THE COMPLETE MEDITERRANEAN DIET COOKBOOK

A Collection of 50 Healthy and Quick Recipes to Enjoy the Flavors of the Mediterranean at Your Table

Healthy & Lovely

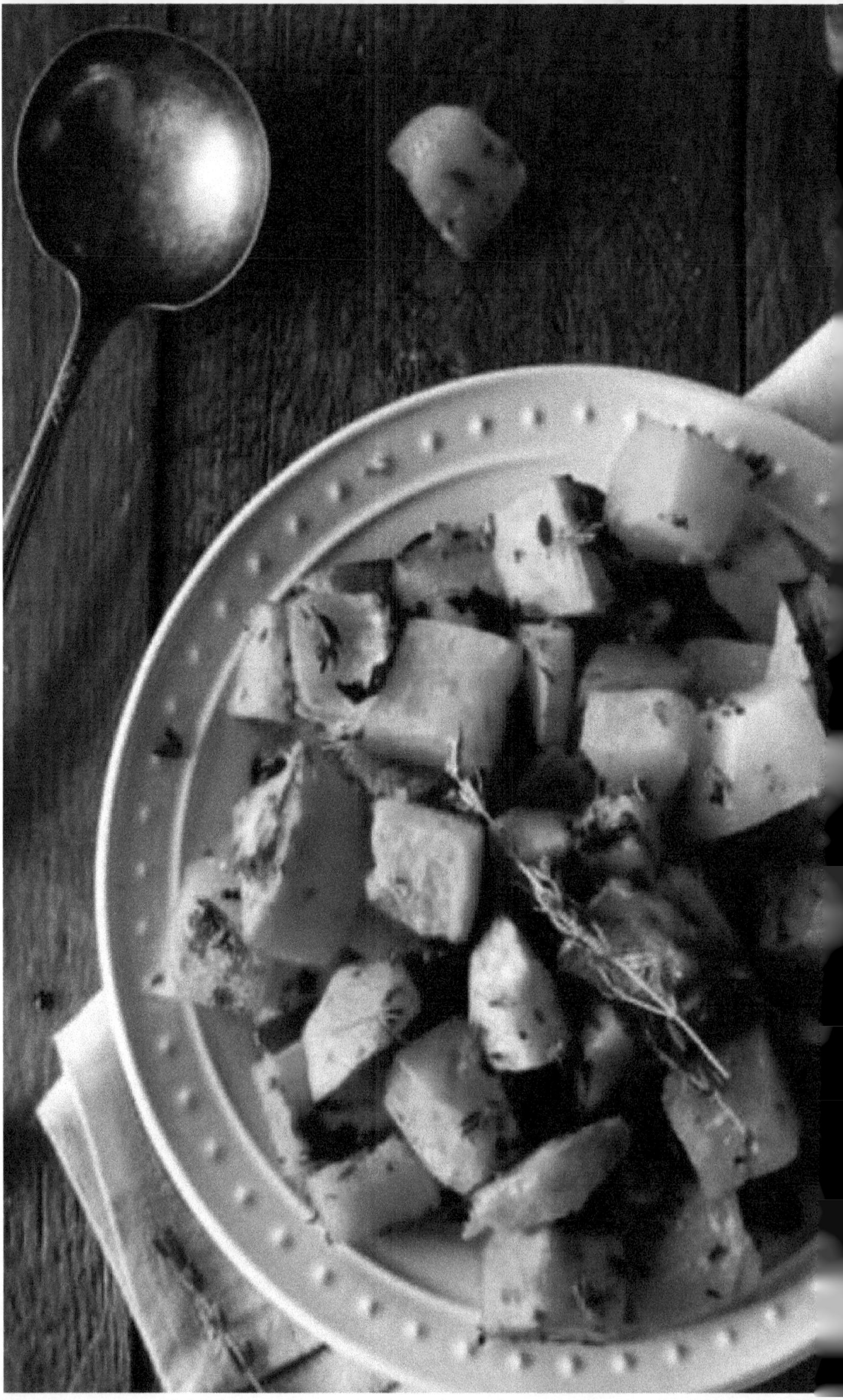

inattention, use, or misuse of the information in question by the reader will render any resulting actions solely under their purview. There are no scenarios in which the publisher or the original author of this work can be in any fashion deemed liable for any hardship or damages that may befall them after undertaking information described herein.

Additionally, the information in the following pages is intended only for informational purposes and should thus be thought of as universal. As befitting its nature, it is presented without assurance regarding its prolonged validity or interim quality. Trademarks that are mentioned are done without written consent and can in no way be considered an endorsement from the trademark holder.

Table of Contents

INTRODUCTION

Mediterranean Diet

A Mediterranean diet incorporates the traditional healthy living habits of people from countries bordering the Mediterranean Sea, including France, Greece, Italy, and Spain. A traditional diet from the Mediterranean region includes a generous portion of fresh produce, whole grains, and legumes, as well as some healthful fats and fish. In general, it's high in vegetables, fruits, legumes, nuts, beans, cereals, grains, fish, and unsaturated fats such as olive oil. It usually includes a low intake of meat and dairy foods.

When you think about Mediterranean food, your mind may go to pizza and pasta from Italy or lamb chops from Greece, but these dishes don't fit into the healthy dietary plans advertised as "Mediterranean." That's how the inhabitants of Crete, Greece, and Southern Italy ate circa 1960, when their rates of chronic disease were among the lowest in the world and their life expectancy among the highest, despite having only limited medical services.

And the real Mediterranean diet is about more than just eating fresh, wholesome food. Daily physical activity and sharing meals with others are vital elements. Together, they can have a profound effect on your mood and mental health and help you foster a deep appreciation for the pleasures of eating healthy and delicious foods.

Of course, making changes to your diet is rarely easy, especially if you're trying to move away from the convenience of processed and takeout foods. But the Mediterranean diet can be an inexpensive as well as a satisfying and very healthy way to eat. Making the switch from pepperoni and pasta to fish and avocados may take some effort, but you could soon be on the path to a healthier and longer life.

If you have a chronic condition like heart disease or high blood pressure, your doctor may even have prescribed it to you. It is often promoted to decrease the risk of heart disease, depression, and dementia.

Research has consistently shown that the Mediterranean diet is effective in reducing the risk of cardiovascular diseases and overall mortality. [3, 4] A study of nearly 26,000 women found that those who followed this type of diet had 25 percent less risk of developing cardiovascular disease over the course of 12 years. [5] The study examined a range of underlying mechanisms that might account for this reduction, and found that changes in inflammation, blood sugar, and body mass index were the biggest drivers.

Tip for Making Your Diet More Mediterranean

You can make your diet more Mediterranean-style by:

- Including fish in your diet
- Choosing products made from vegetable and plant oils, such as olive oil
- Eating plenty of fruit and vegetables
- Eating plenty of starchy foods, such as bread and pasta
- Eating less meat
- Eating less dairy products
- Eating less packaged foods

Avoid the Following Foods If You Are on a Mediterranean Diet

- Foods with added sugars, such as pastries, sodas, and candies
- Refined grains such as white bread, white pasta, and pizza dough containing white flour
- Processed or packaged foods
- Refined oils, which include canola oil and soybean oil
- Deli meats, hot dogs, and other processed meats
- Dairy products

Benefits of Following a Mediterranean Diet

- Can help fight against cancer, diabetes, and cognitive decline
- Reduces the risk of Parkinson's disease
- Increases longevity
- Reduces the risk of Alzheimer's
- Protects against type 2 diabetes
- Prevents heart diseases and strokes
- Keeps you agile

Tips for a Quick Start to a Mediterranean Diet

The easiest way to make the change to a Mediterranean diet is to start with small steps.

You can do this by:

- Limit high-fat dairy by switching to skim or 1% milk.
- Eating more fruits and vegetables by enjoying salad as a starter or side dish, snacking on fruit, and adding veggies to other dishes.
- Choosing whole grains instead of refined breads, rice, and pasta.
- Sautéing food in olive oil instead of butter.
- Substituting fish for red meat at least twice per week.
- Prefer vegetables instead of meat.

1-Week Mediterranean Meal Plan

Breakfast

Greek yogurt with strawberries and oats

Lunch

Whole-grain sandwich with vegetables

Dinner

A tuna salad, dressed in olive oil, fruit for dessert

Tuesday

Breakfast

Oatmeal with raisins

Lunch

Leftover tuna salad from the night before

Dinner

Salad with tomatoes, olives, and feta cheese

Wednesday

Breakfast

Omelet with veggies, tomatoes and onions, a piece of fruit

Lunch

Whole-grain sandwich with cheese and fresh vegetables

Dinner

Mediterranean lasagna

Thursday

Breakfast

Yogurt with sliced fruits and nuts

Lunch

Leftover lasagna

Dinner

Broiled salmon, served with brown rice and vegetables

Friday

Breakfast

Eggs and vegetables fried in olive oil

Lunch

Greek yogurt with strawberries, oats, and nuts

Dinner

Grilled lamb with salad and baked potato

Saturday

Breakfast

Oatmeal with raisins, nuts, and an apple

Lunch

Whole-grain sandwich with vegetables

Dinner

Mediterranean pizza made with whole wheat, topped with cheese, vegetables, and olives

BREAKFAST

Tasty Tofu with Mushrooms

Servings: 4

Preparation Time: 25 minutes

Per Serving: Calories: 423 Fat: 37g Carbohydrates: 4g Protein: 23.1g Sugar: 0.9g Sodium: 691mg

Ingredients:

- 2 Cups fresh mushrooms, chopped finely
- 2 Block tofu, pressed and cubed into 1-inch pieces
- 8 Tablespoons butter
- Salt and black pepper, to taste
- 8 Tablespoons Parmesan cheese, shredded

Procedure:

1. Firstly, season the tofu with salt and black pepper.
2. Then, put butter and seasoned tofu in a pan and cook for about 5 minutes.
3. Add mushrooms and Parmesan cheese and cook for another 5 minutes, stirring occasionally.

4. Now, dish out and serve immediately or refrigerate for about 3 days wrapped in a foil for meal prepping and microwave it to serve again.

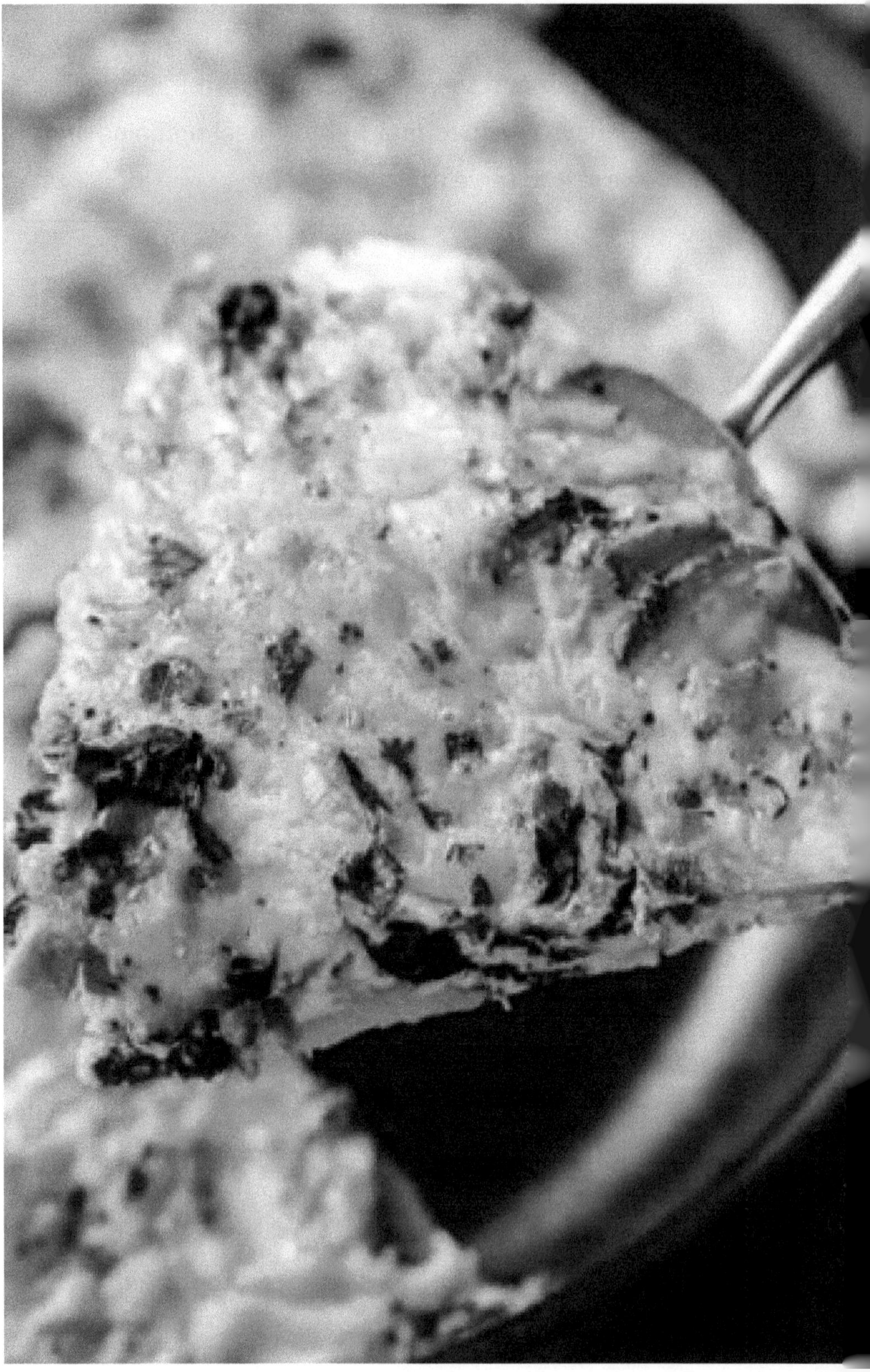

Yummy Ham Spinach Ballet

Servings: 4

Preparation Time: 40 minutes

Per Serving: Calories: 188 Fat: 12.5g Carbohydrates: 4.9g Protein: 14.6g Sugar: 0.3g Sodium: 1098mg

Ingredients:

- 8 Teaspoons cream
- ¾ Pound fresh baby spinach
- 14-Ounce ham, sliced
- Salt and black pepper, to taste
- 2 Tablespoons unsalted butter, melted

Procedure:

1. Firstly, preheat the oven to 360 degrees F. and grease 2 ramekins with butter.
2. Then, put butter and spinach in a skillet and cook for about 3 minutes.
3. Add cooked spinach in the ramekins and top with ham slices, cream, salt and black pepper.

4. Finally, bake for about 25 minutes and dish out to serve hot.

5. Now, for meal prepping, you can refrigerate this ham spinach ballet for about 3 days wrapped in a foil.

Vegetarian Three Cheese Quiche Stuffed Peppers

Servings: 4

Preparation Time: 50 minutes

Per Serving: Calories: 157 Carbs: 7.3g Fats: 9g Proteins: 12.7g Sodium: 166mg Sugar: 3.7g

Ingredients:

- 4 Large eggs
- 1/2 Cup mozzarella, shredded
- 1 Medium bell peppers, sliced in half and seeds removed
- 1/2 Cup ricotta cheese
- 1/2 Cup grated Parmesan cheese
- 1 Teaspoon garlic powder
- 1/4 Cup baby spinach leaves
- 1/2 Teaspoon dried parsley
- 2 Tablespoons Parmesan cheese, to garnish

Procedure:

1. Firstly, preheat oven to 375 degrees F.

2. Then, blend all the cheeses, eggs, garlic powder and parsley in a food processor and process until smooth.
3. Pour the cheese mixture into each sliced bell pepper and top with spinach leaves.
4. Stir with a fork, pushing them under the cheese mixture and cover with foil.
5. Finally, bake for about 40 minutes and sprinkle with Parmesan cheese.
6. Now, broil for about 5 minutes and dish out to serve.

Delightful Spinach Artichoke Egg Casserole

Servings: 4

Preparation Time: 45 minutes

Per Serving: Calories: 228 Carbs: 10.1g Fats: 13.3g Proteins: 19.1g Sodium: 571mg Sugar: 2.5g

Ingredients:

- 1/4 Cup milk
- 5-Ounce frozen chopped spinach, thawed and drained well
- 1/4 Cup parmesan cheese
- 1/4 Cup onions, shaved
- 1/2 Teaspoon salt
- 1/2 Teaspoon crushed red pepper
- 8 Large eggs
- 7-Ounce artichoke hearts, drained
- 1/2 Cup white cheddar, shredded
- 1/4 Cup ricotta cheese
- 1 Garlic clove, minced
- 1/2 Teaspoon dried thyme

Procedure:

1. Firstly, preheat the oven to 350 degrees F and grease a baking dish with non-stick cooking spray.
2. Whisk eggs and milk together and add artichoke hearts and spinach.
3. Then, mix well and stir in the rest of the ingredients, withholding the ricotta cheese.
4. Pour the mixture into the baking dish and top evenly with ricotta cheese.
5. Transfer in the oven and bake for about 30 minutes.
6. Now, dish out and serve warm.

Quick Cream of Wheat

Servings: 2

Preparation Time: 10 minutes

Per Serving:

Ingredients:

- 8 Cups whole milk
- 1 Cup farina
- 1 Tsp salt
- 6 Tsps sugar
- 6 Tsps butter
- 6 Tsps pine nuts

Procedure:

1. Firstly, in a large saucepan over medium heat, bring whole milk to a simmer, and cook for about 4 minutes. Do not allow milk to scorch.
2. Then, whisk in farina, salt, and sugar, and bring to a slight boil. Cook for 2 minutes, reduce heat to low and cook for 3 more minutes. Stay close to the pan to ensure it doesn't boil over.

3. Finally, pour the mixture into 4 bowls, and let cool for 5 minutes.
4. Meanwhile, in a small pan over low heat, cook butter and pine nuts for about 3 minutes or until pine nuts are lightly toasted.
5. Now, evenly spoon butter and pine nuts over each bowl, and serve warm.

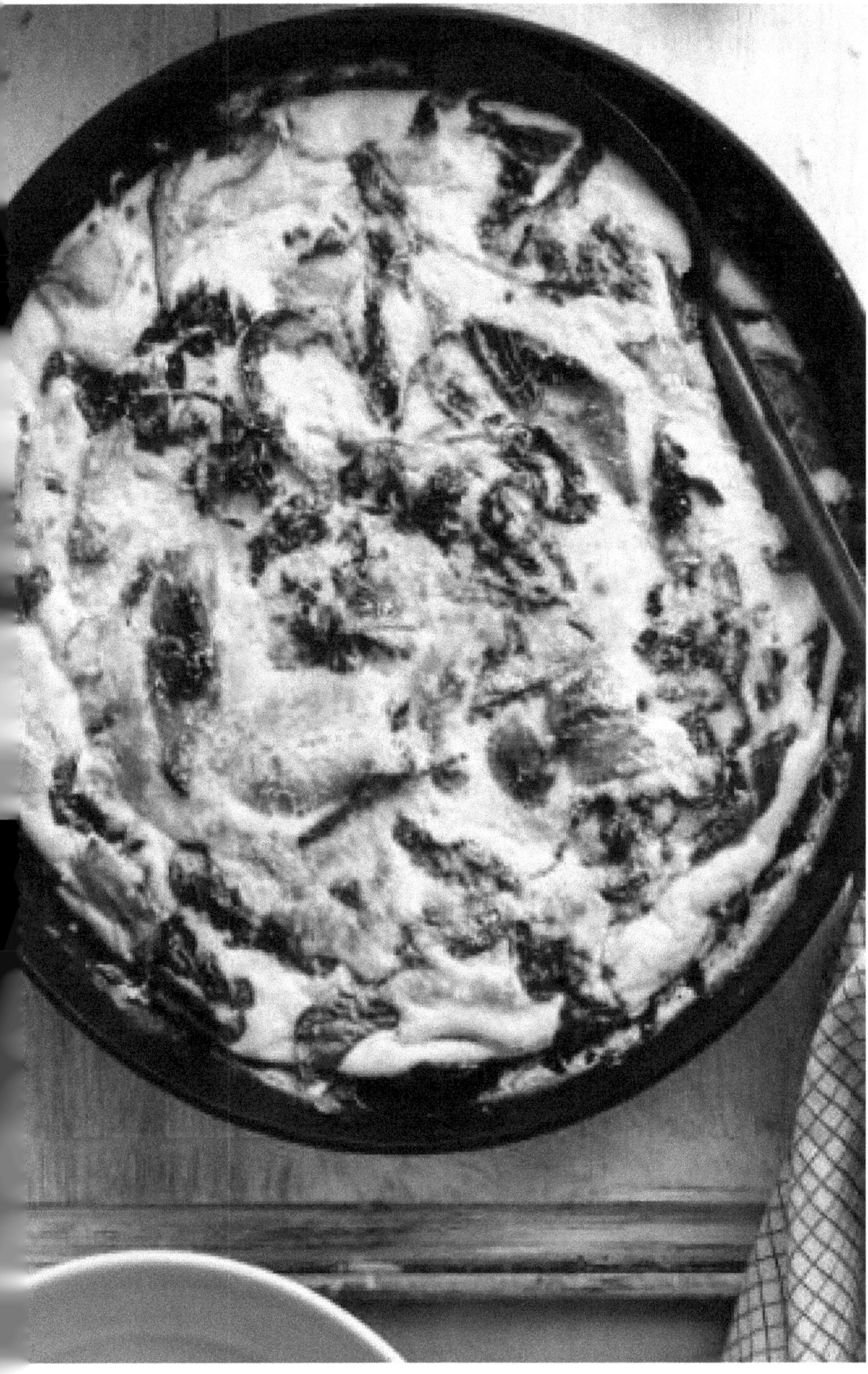

Pleasant Herbed Spinach Frittata

Servings: 8

Preparation Time: 20 minutes

Per Serving: calories 140, fat 9.8, fiber 0.5, carbs 2.1, protein 11.9

Ingredients:

- 10 Eggs, beaten
- 1 Cup fresh spinach
- 4 Oz Parmesan, grated
- 1 Cup cherry tomatoes
- 1 Teaspoon dried oregano
- 2 Teaspoons dried thyme
- 2 Teaspoons olive oil

Procedure:

1. Firstly, chop the spinach into tiny pieces and or use a blender.
2. Then, combine together chopped spinach with eggs, dried oregano and thyme.

3. Add Parmesan and stir frittata mixture with the help of the fork.
4. Brush the springform pan with olive oil and pour the egg mixture inside.
5. Cut the cherry tomatoes into halves and place them over the egg mixture.
6. Finally, preheat the oven to 360F.
7. Bake the frittata for 20 minutes or until it is solid.
8. Now, chill the cooked breakfast till room temperature and slice it into the servings.

Tempting Banana Quinoa

Servings: 8

Preparation Time: 10 minutes

Per Serving: Calories 279, fat 5.3, fiber 4.6, carbs 48.4, protein 10.7

Ingredients:

- 2 Cups quinoa
- 4 Cups milk
- 2 Teaspoons vanilla extract
- 2 Teaspoons honey
- 4 Bananas, sliced
- 1/2 Teaspoon ground cinnamon

Procedure:

1. Firstly, pour milk in the saucepan and add quinoa.
2. Then, close the lid and cook it over medium heat for 12 minutes or until quinoa will absorb all liquid.
3. Finally, chill the quinoa for 10-15 minutes and place it in the serving mason jars.
4. Add honey, vanilla extract, and ground cinnamon.
5. Stir well.
6. Now, top quinoa with banana and stir it before serving.

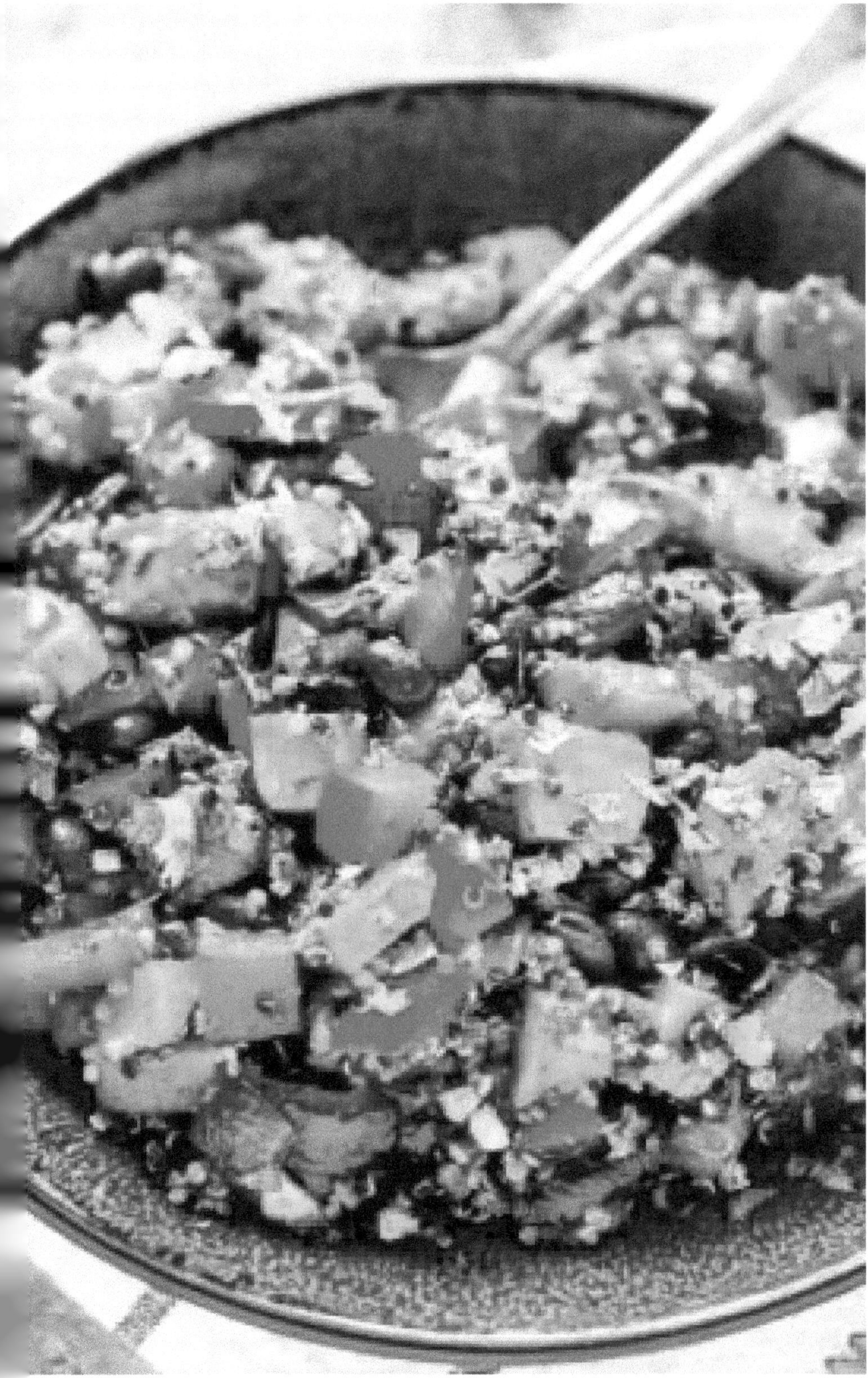

Enticing Quinoa and Potato Bowl

Servings: 8

Preparation Time: 20 minutes

Per Serving: calories 221, fat 7.1, fiber 3.9, carbs 33.2, protein 6.6

Ingredients:

- 2 Sweet potatoes, peeled, chopped
- 2 Tablespoons olive oil
- 1 Teaspoon chili flakes
- 1 Teaspoon salt
- 1 Cup quinoa
- 2 Cups of water
- 2 Teaspoons butter
- 2 Tablespoons fresh cilantro, chopped

Procedure:

1. Firstly, line the baking tray with parchment.
2. Then, arrange the chopped sweet potato in the tray and sprinkle it with chili flakes, salt, and olive oil.
3. Bake the sweet potato for 20 minutes at 355F.

4. Meanwhile, pour water in the saucepan.
5. Add quinoa and cook it over medium heat for 7 minutes or until quinoa will absorb all liquid.
6. Finally, add butter in the cooked quinoa and stir well.
7. Now, transfer it in the bowls, add baked sweet potato and chopped cilantro.

Tasty Tomato and Egg Breakfast Pizza

Servings: 4

Preparation Time: 20 minutes

Per Serving: calories: 429 | fat: 16.8g | protein: 18.1g | carbs: 12.0g | fiber: 4.8g | sodium: 682mg

Ingredients:

- 4 (6- to 8-inch-long) slices of whole-wheat naan bread
- 4 Tablespoons prepared pesto
- 2 Medium tomatoes, sliced
- 4 Large eggs

Procedure:

1. First, heat a large non-stick skillet over medium-high heat. Place the naan bread in the skillet and let warm for about 2 minutes on each side or until softened.
2. Then, spread 1 tablespoon of the pesto on one side of each slice and top with tomato slices.
3. Remove from the skillet and place each one on its own plate.

4. Crack the eggs into the skillet, keeping them separated, and cook until the whites are no longer translucent and the yolk is cooked to desired doneness.
5. Now, using a spatula, spoon one egg onto each bread slice. Serve warm.

Yummy Classic Shakshuka

Servings: 4

Preparation Time: 45 minutes

Per Serving: calories: 289 | fat: 18.2g | protein: 15.1g | carbs: 18.5g | fiber: 4.9g | sodium: 432mg

Ingredients:

- 2 Tablespoons olive oil
- 1 Red pepper, diced
- 1 Medium onion, diced
- 4 Small garlic cloves, minced
- 1 Teaspoon smoked paprika
- 1 Teaspoon cumin
- Pinch red pepper flakes
- 2 (14.5-ounce / 411-g) can fire-roasted tomatoes
- 1/2 teaspoon salt
- Pinch freshly ground black pepper
- 2 ounce (28 g) crumbled feta cheese (about ¼ cup)
- 6 Large eggs
- 6 Tablespoons minced fresh parsley

Procedure:

1. Firstly, heat the olive oil in a skillet over medium-high heat and add the pepper, onion, and garlic.
2. Sauté until the vegetables start to turn golden.
3. Then, add the paprika, cumin, and red pepper flakes and stir to toast the spices for about 30 seconds.
4. Add the tomatoes with their juices.
5. Reduce the heat and let the sauce simmer for 10 minutes or until it starts to thicken.
6. Add the salt and pepper.
7. Taste the sauce and adjust seasonings as necessary.
8. Scatter the feta cheese on top. Make 3 wells in the sauce and crack one egg into each well.
9. Cover and let the eggs cook for about 7 minutes.
10. Finally, remove the lid and continue cooking for 5 minutes more, or until the yolks are cooked to desired doneness.
11. Now, garnish with fresh parsley and serve.

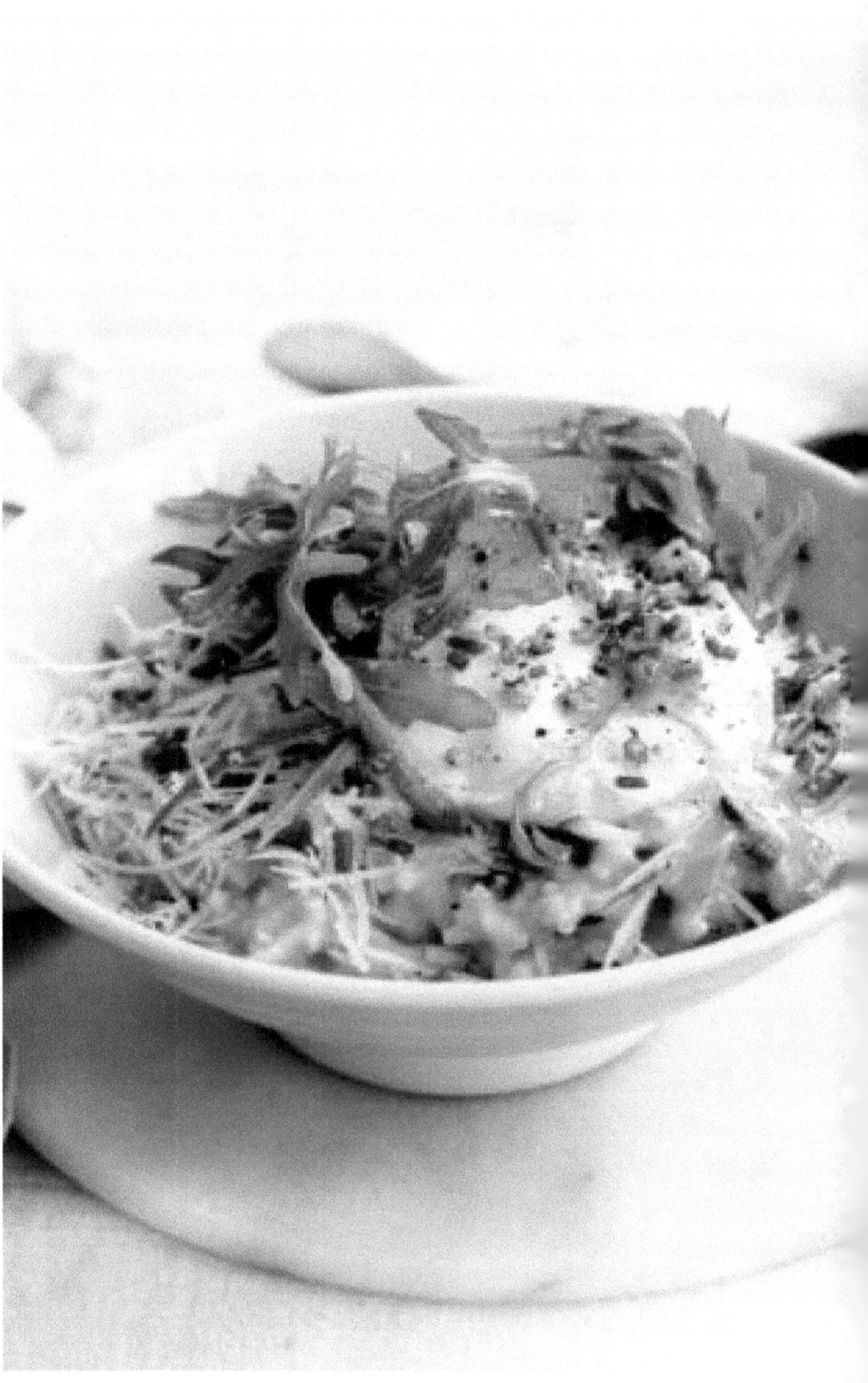

Tempting Parmesan Oatmeal with Greens

Servings: 4

Preparation Time: 20 minutes

Per Serving: calories: 257 | fat: 14.0g | protein: 12.2g | carbs: 30.2g | fiber: 6.1g | sodium: 262mg

Ingredients:

- 2 Tablespoons olive oil
- 1/2 Cup minced onion
- 4 Cups greens (arugula, baby spinach, chopped kale, or Swiss chard)
- ¾ Cup gluten-free old-fashioned oats
- 3 Cups water, or low-sodium chicken stock
- 4 Tablespoons Parmesan cheese
- Salt, to taste
- Pinch freshly ground black pepper

Procedure:

1. Firstly, heat the olive oil in a saucepan over medium-high heat.

2. Then, add the minced onion and sauté for 2 minutes, or until softened.
3. Add the greens and stir until they begin to wilt. Transfer this mixture to a bowl and set aside.
4. Add the oats to the pan and let them toast for about 2 minutes. Add the water and bring the oats to a boil.
5. Reduce the heat to low, cover, and let the oats cook for 10 minutes, or until the liquid is absorbed and the oats are tender.
6. Stir the Parmesan cheese into the oats, and add the onion and greens back to the pan.
7. Finally, add additional water if needed, so the oats are creamy and not dry.
8. Now, stir well and season with salt and black pepper to taste. Serve warm.

Delectable Mediterranean Omelet

Servings: 4

Preparation Time: 25 minutes

Per Serving: calories: 206 | fat: 14.2g | protein: 13.7g | carbs: 7.2g | fiber: 1.2g | sodium: 729mg

Ingredients:

- 4 Teaspoons extra-virgin olive oil, divided
- 1 Garlic clove, minced
- 1 Yellow bell pepper, thinly sliced
- 1 Red bell pepper, thinly sliced
- 1/2 Cup thinly sliced red onion
- 4 Tablespoons chopped fresh parsley, plus extra for garnish
- 4 Tablespoons chopped fresh basil
- 1 Teaspoon salt
- 1 Teaspoon freshly ground black pepper
- 8 Large eggs, beaten

Procedure:

1. Firstly, in a large, heavy skillet, heat 1 teaspoon of the olive oil over medium heat.
2. Then, add the garlic, peppers, and onion to the skillet and sauté, stirring frequently, for 5 minutes.
3. Add the parsley, basil, salt, and pepper, increase the heat to medium-high, and sauté for 2 minutes.
4. Slide the vegetable mixture onto a plate and return the skillet to the heat.
5. Heat the remaining 1 teaspoon of olive oil in the skillet and pour in the beaten eggs, tilting the pan to coat evenly.
6. Cook the eggs just until the edges are bubbly and all but the center is dry, 3 to 5 minutes.
7. Spoon the vegetable mixture onto one-half of the omelet and use a spatula to fold the empty side over the top.
8. Finally, slide the omelet onto a platter or cutting board.
9. Now, to serve, cut the omelet in half and garnish with extra fresh parsley.

Easy Berry and Nut Parfait

Servings: 4

Preparation Time: 10 minutes

Per Serving: calories: 507 | fat: 23.0g | protein: 24.1g | carbs: 57.0g | fiber: 8.2g | sodium: 172mg

Ingredients:

- 4 Cups plain Greek yogurt
- 4 Tablespoons honey
- 2 Cups fresh raspberries
- 2 Cups fresh blueberries
- 1 Cup walnut pieces

Procedure:

1. Firstly, in a medium bowl, whisk the yogurt and honey. Spoon into 2 serving bowls.
2. Then, top each with ½ cup blueberries, ½ cup raspberries, and ¼ cup walnut pieces. Serve immediately.

MAIN DISHES

Tasty Cauliflower Tomato Beef

Servings: 4

Preparation Time: 35 minutes

Per Serving: Calories 306 Fat 14.3 g Carbohydrates 7.6 g Sugar 3.5 g Protein 35.7 g Cholesterol 101 mg

Ingredients:

- 1 lb beef stew meat, chopped
- 2 Tsps paprika
- 2 Tbsps balsamic vinegar
- 2 Celery stalks, chopped
- 1 Cup grape tomatoes, chopped
- 2 Onions, chopped
- 2 Tbsps olive oil
- 1/2 Cup cauliflower, chopped
- Pepper
- Salt

Procedure:

1. Firstly, add oil into the instant pot and set the pot on sauté mode.

2. Then, add meat and sauté for 5 minutes.

3. Add remaining ingredients and stir well.

4. Finally, seal the pot with a lid and cook on high for 20 minutes.

5. Once done, allow to release pressure naturally. Remove lid.

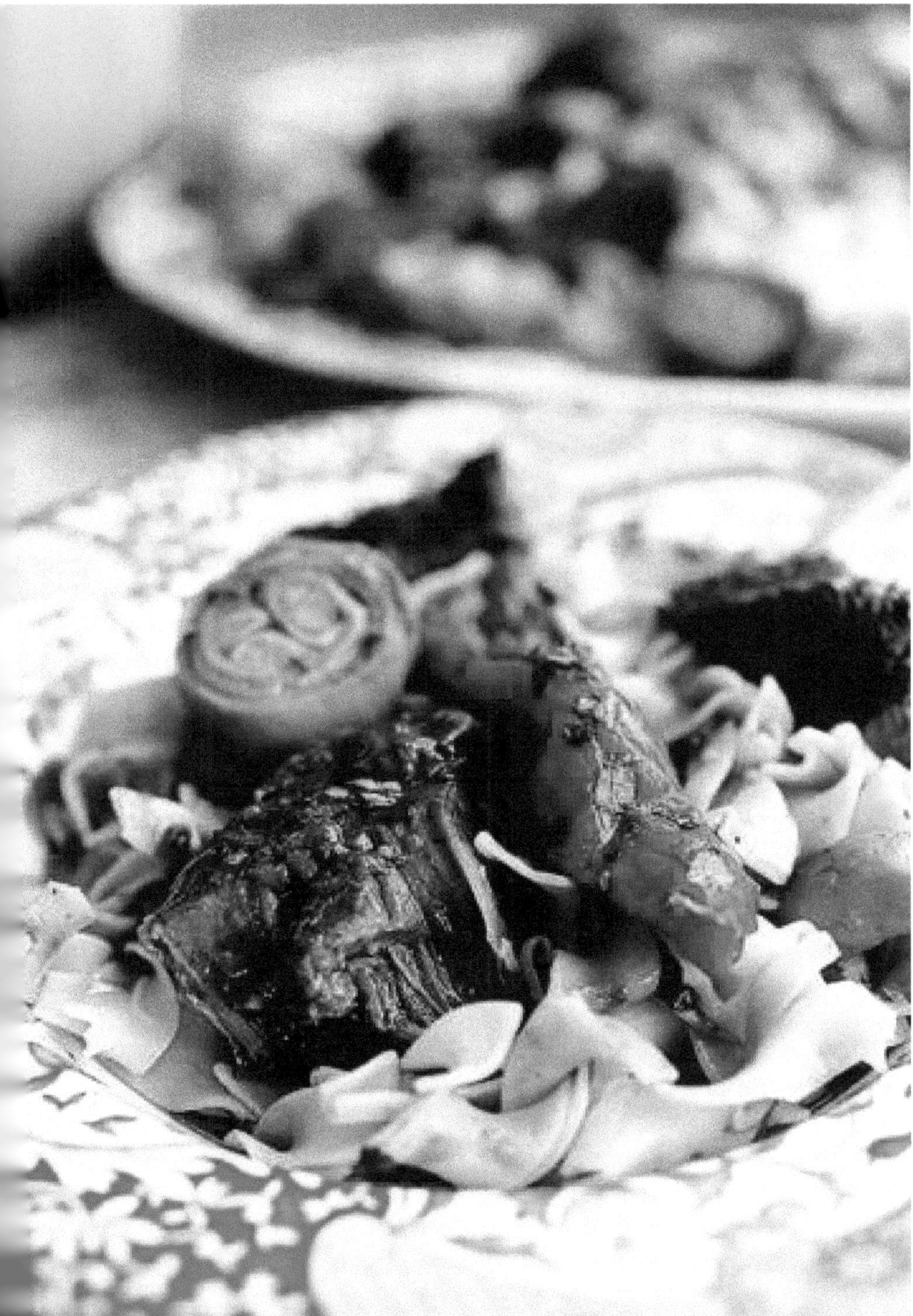

Yummy Artichoke Beef Roast

Servings: 12

Preparation Time: 55 minutes

Per Serving: Calories 344 Fat 12.2 g Carbohydrates 9.2 g Sugar 2.6 g Protein 48.4 g Cholesterol 135 mg

Ingredients:

- 4 lbs beef roast, cubed
- 2 Tbsps garlic, minced
- 1 Onion, chopped
- 1 Tsp paprika
- 2 Tbsps parsley, chopped
- 4 Tomatoes, chopped
- 12 Tbsps capers, chopped
- 20 Oz can artichokes, drained and chopped
- 4 Cups chicken stock
- 2 Tbsps olive oil
- Pepper
- Salt

Procedure:

1. Firstly, add oil into the instant pot and set the pot on sauté mode.
2. Then, add garlic and onion and sauté for 5 minutes.
3. Add meat and cook until brown.
4. Add remaining ingredients and stir well.
5. Finally, seal pot with lid and cook on high for 35 minutes.
6. Once done, allow to release pressure naturally. Remove lid.
7. Now, serve and enjoy.

Tasty Beanless Beef Chili

Servings: 8

Preparation Time: 30 minutes

Per Serving: Calories 387 Fat 22.2 g Carbohydrates 9.5 g Sugar 5 g Protein 37.2 g Cholesterol 142 mg

Ingredients:

- 2 lbs ground beef
- 1 Tsp dried rosemary
- 1 Tsp paprika
- 2 Tsps garlic powder
- 1Tsp chili powder
- 1 Cup chicken broth
- 2 Cups heavy cream
- 2 Tbsps olive oil
- 2 Tsps garlic, minced
- 2 Small onions, chopped
- 2 Bell peppers, chopped
- 4 Cups tomatoes, diced
- Pepper
- Salt

Procedure:

1. Firstly, add oil into the instant pot and set the pot on sauté mode.
2. Add meat, bell pepper, and onion and sauté for 5 minutes.
3. Then, add the remaining ingredients except for heavy cream and stir well.
4. Seal pot with lid and cook on high for 5 minutes.
5. Once done, release pressure using quick release. Remove lid.
6. Finally, add heavy cream and stir well and cook on sauté mode for 10 minutes.
7. Now, serve and enjoy.

Delicious Spicy Tomato Poached Eggs

Servings: 8

Preparation Time: 30 minutes

Per Serving: Calories:179 Fat:11.9g Protein:7.6g Carbohydrates:11.7g

Ingredients:

- 4 Tablespoons olive oil
- 4 Shallots, chopped
- 4 Garlic cloves, chopped
- 4 Red bell peppers, cored and sliced
- 4 yellow bell peppers, cored and sliced
- 4 Tomatoes, peeled and diced
- 2 Cups vegetable stock
- 2 Jalapenos, chopped
- Salt and pepper to taste
- 8 Eggs

Procedure:

1. Firstly, heat the oil in a saucepan and stir in the shallots, garlic, bell peppers and jalapeno. Cook for 5 minutes.

2. Then, add the tomatoes, stock, thyme and bay leaf, as well as salt and pepper to taste.
3. Cook for 10 minutes on low heat.
4. Crack open the eggs and drop them in the hot sauce.
5. Finally, cook on low heat for 5 additional minutes.
6. Now, serve the eggs and the sauce fresh and warm.

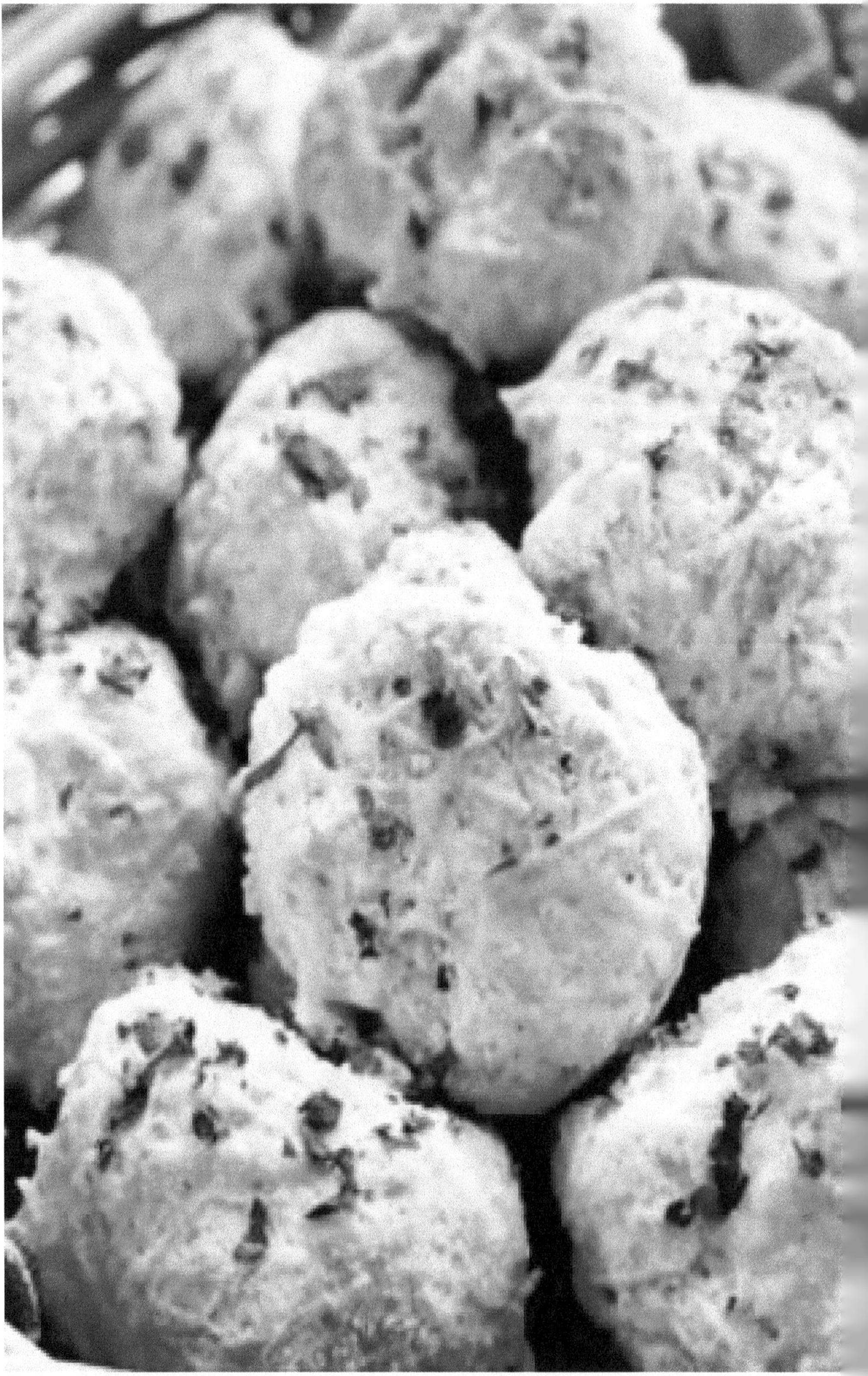

Pleasant Mediterranean Scones

Servings: 4

Preparation Time: 20 minutes

Per Serving: 293 Cal, 14 g total fat (7 g sat. fat), 36 g carb.,0 g sugar, 2 g fiber, 8 g protein, and 2 g sodium.

Ingredients:

- 1/2 Egg, beaten, to glaze
- 1/2 Tablespoon baking powder
- 1/2 Tablespoon olive oil
- 1/8 Tsp salt
- 5 Black olives, pitted, halved
- 50 g Feta cheese, cubed
- 150 Ml full-fat milk
- 350 Gself-rising whole-wheat flour
- 25 G butter, cut in pieces
- 4 Halves Italian sundried tomatoes, coarsely chopped

Procedure:

1. Firstly, preheat the oven to 220C, gas to 7, or fan to 200C.

2. Grease a large-sized baking sheet with butter.
3. Then, in a large mixing bowl, mix the flour, the baking powder, and the salt. Rub in the oil and the butter, until the flour mix resembles fine crumbs.
4. Add the cheese, tomatoes, and the olives.
5. Finally, create a well in the center of the flour mix, pour the milk, and with a knife, mix using cutting movements until the flour mixture is a stickyish, soft dough.
6. Make sure that you do not over mix the dough.
7. Flour the work surface and your hands well; shape the dough into 3 to 4-cm think round.
8. Cut into 8 wedges; place the wedges well apart in the prepared baking sheet. Brush the wedges with the beaten egg; bake for about 15-20 minutes until the dough has risen, golden, and springy.
9. Transfer into a wire rack; cover with a clean tea towel to keep them soft.
10. Now, serve warm and buttered.
11. Store in an airtight container for up to 2 to 3 days.

Easy Mixed Olives Braised Chicken

Servings: 8

Preparation Time: 1 hour

Per Serving: Calories:280 Fat:16.3g Protein:22.9g Carbohydrates:7.9g

Ingredients:

- 8 Chicken breasts
- 4 Shallots, sliced
- 8 garlic cloves, chopped
- 4 Red bell peppers, cored and sliced
- 1 Cup black olives
- 1 Cup green olives
- 1 Cup kalamata olives
- 4 Tablespoons olive oil
- 1/2 Cup white wine
- 1 Cup vegetable stock
- Salt and pepper to taste
- 1 Bay leaf
- 2 Thyme sprig

Procedure:

1. First, combine the shallots, garlic, bell peppers, olives, oil, wine and stock in a deep dish baking pan.
2. Then, season with salt and pepper and place the chicken in the pan over the olives.
3. Cook in the preheated oven at 350F for 45 minutes.
4. Now, serve the chicken warm and fresh.

Tasty Coconut Chicken Meatballs

Servings: 8

Preparation Time: 10 minutes

Per Serving: calories 200, fat 11.5, fiber 0.6, carbs 1.7, protein 21.9

Ingredients:

- 4 Cups ground chicken
- 2 Teaspoons minced garlic
- 2 Teaspoons dried dill
- 1 Carrot, grated
- 2 Eggs, beaten
- 2 Tablespoons olive oil
- 1/2 Cup coconut flakes
- 1 Teaspoon salt

Procedure:

1. Firstly, in the mixing bowl, mix up together ground chicken, minced garlic, dried dill, carrot, egg, and salt.
2. Then, stir the chicken mixture with the help of the fingertips until homogenous.

3. Finally, make medium balls from the mixture.
4. Coat every chicken ball in coconut flakes.
5. Heat up olive oil in the skillet.
6. Add chicken balls and cook them for 3 minutes from each side.
7. Now, cooked chicken balls will have a golden brown color.

Yummy Grilled Turkey with White Beans Mash

Servings: 8

Preparation Time: 45 minutes

Per Serving: Calories:337 Fat:8.2g Protein:21.1g Carbohydrates:47.2g

Ingredients:

- 8 turkey breast fillets
- 2 Teaspoons chili powder
- 1 Teaspoon dried parsley
- Salt and pepper to taste
- 4 Cans white beans, drained
- 8 Garlic cloves, minced
- 4 Tablespoons lemon juice
- 6 tablespoons olive oil
- 4 Sweet onions, sliced
- 4 Tablespoons tomato paste

Procedure:

1. Firstly, season the turkey with salt, pepper and dried parsley.

2. Heat a grill pan over medium flame and place the turkey on the grill. Cook on each side for 7 minutes.
3. For the mash, combine the beans, garlic, lemon juice, salt and pepper in a blender and pulse until well mixed and smooth.
4. Then, heat the oil in a skillet and add the onions. Cook for 10 minutes until caramelized.
5. Add the tomato paste and cook for 2 more minutes.
6. Now, serve the grilled turkey with bean mash and caramelized onions.

Easy Sauteed Cabbage with Parsley

Servings: 12

Preparation Time: 15 minutes

Per Serving: calories: 117 | fat: 7.0g | protein: 2.7g | carbs: 13.4g | fiber: 5.1g | sodium: 472mg

Ingredients:

- 2 Small head green cabbages (about 1¼ pounds / 567 g), cored and sliced thin
- 4 Tablespoons extra-virgin olive oil, divided
- 2 Onions, halved and sliced thin
- ¾ Teaspoon salt, divided
- 1/2 Teaspoon black pepper
- 1 Cup chopped fresh parsley
- 1 Teaspoon lemon juice

Procedure:

1. Firstly, place the cabbage in a large bowl with cold water. Let sit for 3 minutes. Drain well.
2. Heat 1 tablespoon of the oil in a skillet over medium-high heat until shimmering.

3. Then, add the onion and ¼ teaspoon of the salt and cook for 5 to 7 minutes, or until softened and lightly browned. Transfer to a bowl.
4. Heat the remaining 1 tablespoon of the oil in a now-empty skillet over medium-high heat until shimmering.
5. Add the cabbage and sprinkle with the remaining ½ teaspoon of the salt and black pepper.
6. Cover and cook for about 3 minutes, without stirring, or until cabbage is wilted and lightly browned on the bottom.
7. Finally, stir and continue to cook for about 4 minutes, uncovered, or until the cabbage is crisp-tender and lightly browned in places, stirring once halfway through cooking.
8. Off heat, stir in the cooked onion, parsley and lemon juice.
9. Now, transfer to a plate and serve.

Flavorful Braised Cauliflower with White Wine

Servings: 12

Preparation Time: 15 minutes

Per Serving: calories: 143 | fat: 11.7g | protein: 3.1g | carbs: 8.7g | fiber: 3.1g | sodium: 263mg

Ingredients:

- 6 Tablespoons plus 1 teaspoon extra-virgin olive oil, divided
- 6 Garlic cloves, minced
- 1/4 Teaspoon red pepper flakes
- 2 Heads cauliflower (2 pounds / 907 g), cored and cut into 3-inch florets
- 1/2 Teaspoon salt, plus more for seasoning
- Black pepper, to taste
- 1 Cup vegetable broth
- 1 Cup dry white wine
- 4 Tablespoons minced fresh parsley

Procedure:

1. Firstly, combine 1 teaspoon of the oil, garlic and pepper flakes in a small bowl.
2. Heat the remaining 3 tablespoons of the oil in a skillet over medium-high heat until shimmering.
3. Then, add the cauliflower and ¼ teaspoon of the salt and cook for 7 to 9 minutes, stirring occasionally, or until florets are golden brown.
4. Push the cauliflower to the sides of the skillet. Add the garlic mixture to the center of the skillet.
5. Cook for about 30 seconds, or until fragrant.
6. Stir the garlic mixture into the cauliflower.
7. Pour in the broth and wine and bring to simmer. Reduce the heat to medium-low.
8. Cover and cook for 4 to 6 minutes, or until the cauliflower is crisp-tender. Off heat, stir in the parsley and season with salt and pepper.
9. Now, serve immediately.

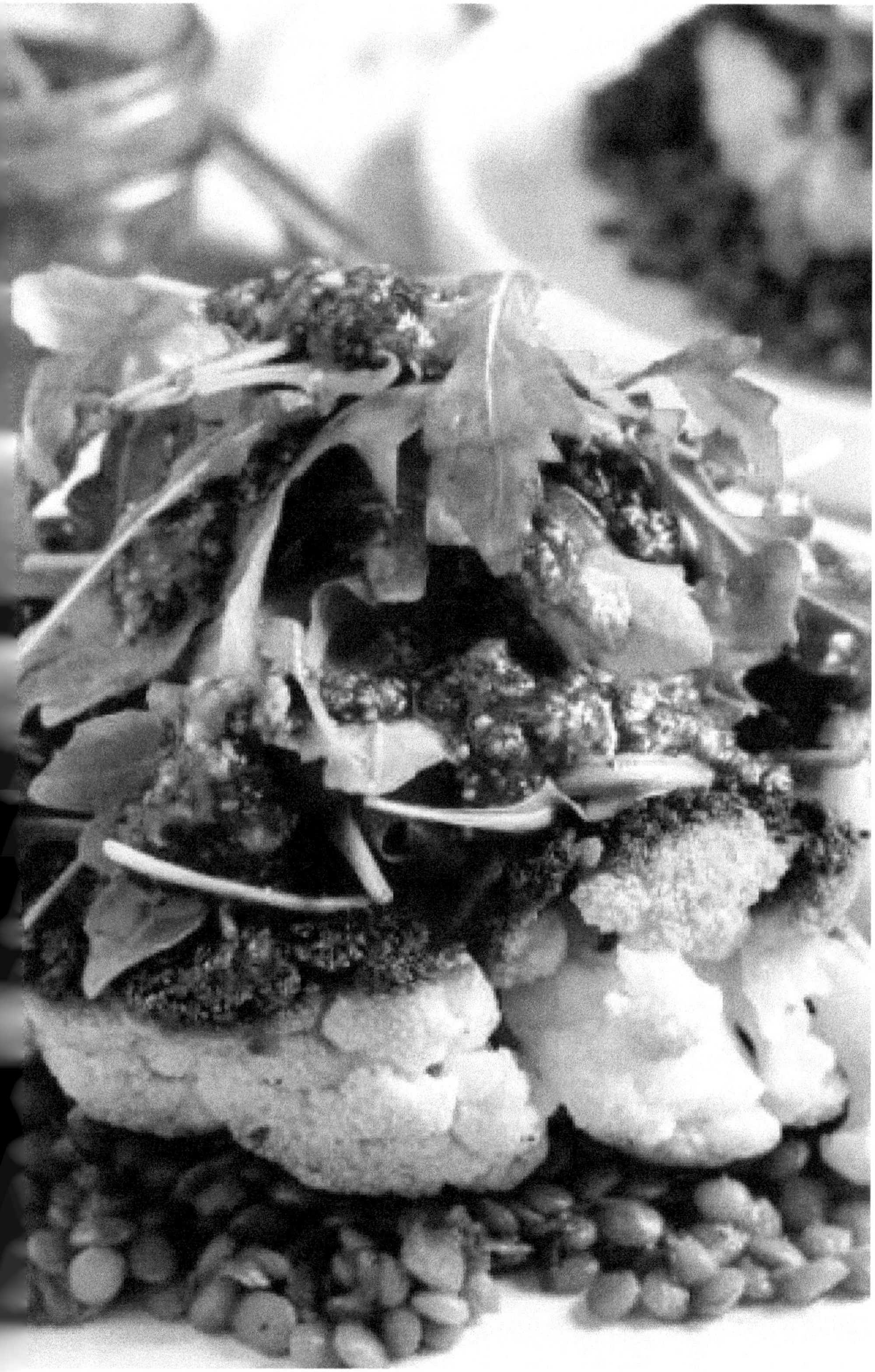

Pleasant Cauliflower Steaks with Arugula

Servings: 8

Preparation Time: 25 minutes

Per Serving: calories: 115 | fat: 6.0g | protein: 5.0g | carbs: 14.0g | fiber: 4.0g | sodium: 97mg

Ingredients:

- 2 Heads cauliflower
- Cooking spray
- 1 Teaspoon garlic powder
- 8 cups arugula
- Dressing:
- 3 Tablespoons extra-virgin olive oil
- 3 Tablespoons honey mustard
- 2 Teaspoons freshly squeezed lemon juice

Procedure:

1. Firstly, preheat the oven to 425ºF (220ºC).
2. Remove the leaves from the cauliflower head, and cut it in half lengthwise. Cut 1½-inch-thick steaks from each half.

3. Then, spritz both sides of each steak with cooking spray and season both sides with garlic powder.
4. Place the cauliflower steaks on a baking sheet, cover with foil, and roast in the oven for 10 minutes.
5. Remove the baking sheet from the oven and gently pull back the foil to avoid the steam.
6. Finally, flip the steaks, then roast uncovered for 10 minutes more.
7. Meanwhile, make the dressing: Whisk together the olive oil, honey mustard and lemon juice in a small bowl.
8. When the cauliflower steaks are done, divide into four equal portions.
9. Top each portion with one-quarter of the arugula and dressing.
10. Now, serve immediately.

Tasty Zoodles with Walnut Pesto

Servings: 8

Preparation Time: 10 minutes

Per Serving: calories: 166 | fat: 16.0g | protein: 4.0g | carbs: 3.0g | fiber: 2.0g | sodium: 307mg

Ingredients:

- 4 Medium zucchinis, spiralized
- ½ Cup extra-virgin olive oil, divided
- 2 Teaspoons minced garlic, divided
- 1 Teaspoon crushed red pepper
- 1/2 Teaspoon freshly ground black pepper, divided
- 1/2 Teaspoon kosher salt, divided
- 4 Tablespoons grated Parmesan cheese, divided
- 2 Cups packed fresh basil leaves
- ¾ Cup walnut pieces, divided

Procedure:

1. Firstly, in a large bowl, stir together the zoodles, 1 tablespoon of the olive oil, ½ teaspoon of the minced

garlic, red pepper, ⅛ teaspoon of the black pepper and ⅛ teaspoon of the salt. Set aside.

2. Then, heat ½ tablespoon of the oil in a large skillet over medium-high heat.

3. Add half of the zoodles to the skillet and cook for 5 minutes, stirring constantly.

4. Finally, transfer the cooked zoodles into a bowl. Repeat with another ½ tablespoon of the oil and the remaining zoodles.

5. When done, add the cooked zoodles to the bowl.

6. Make the pesto: In a food processor, combine the remaining ½ teaspoon of the minced garlic, ⅛ teaspoon of the black pepper and ⅛ teaspoon of the salt, 1 tablespoon of the Parmesan, basil leaves and ¼ cup of the walnuts.

7. Pulse until smooth, and then slowly drizzle the remaining 2 tablespoons of the oil into the pesto. Pulse again until well combined.

8. Add the pesto to the zoodles along with the remaining 1 tablespoon of the Parmesan and the remaining ½ cup of the walnuts.

9. Toss to coat well.

10. Now, serve immediately.

Easy Cheesy Sweet Potato Burger

Servings: 8

Preparation Time: 10 minutes

Per Serving: calories: 290 | fat: 12.0g | protein: 12.0g | carbs: 43.0g | fiber: 8.0g | sodium: 566mg

Ingredients:

- 2 Large sweet potatoes (about 8 ounces / 227 g)
- 4 Tablespoons extra-virgin olive oil, divided
- 2 Cups chopped onion
- 1 Large egg
- 2 Garlic cloves
- 2 Cups old-fashioned rolled oats
- 2 Tablespoons dried oregano
- 2 Tablespoons balsamic vinegar
- ½ Teaspoon kosher salt
- 1 Cup crumbled Gorgonzola cheese

Procedure:

1. Firstly, using a fork, pierce the sweet potato all over and microwave on high for 4 to 5 minutes, until softened in the center. Cool slightly before slicing in half.
2. Meanwhile, in a large skillet over medium-high heat, heat 1 tablespoon of the olive oil. Add the onion and sauté for 5 minutes.
3. Then, spoon the sweet potato flesh out of the skin and put the flesh in a food processor.
4. Add the cooked onion, egg, garlic, oats, oregano, vinegar and salt. Pulse until smooth.
5. Finally, add the cheese and pulse four times to barely combine.
6. Form the mixture into four burgers. Place the burgers on a plate, and press to flatten each to about ¾-inch thick.
7. Wipe out the skillet with a paper towel. Heat the remaining 1 tablespoon of the oil over medium-high heat for about 2 minutes.
8. Add the burgers to the hot oil, then reduce the heat to medium. Cook the burgers for 5 minutes per side.
9. Now, transfer the burgers to a plate and serve.

SNACKS

Enjoyable Spicy Chicken Dip

Servings: 5

Preparation Time: 25 minutes

Per Serving: Calories 248 Fat 19 g Carbohydrates 1.6 g Sugar 0.3 g Protein 17.4 g Cholesterol 83 mg

Ingredients:

- 1/2 lb chicken breast, skinless and boneless
- 1/4 Cup sour cream
- 4 Oz cheddar cheese, shredded
- 1/4 Cup chicken stock
- 1 Jalapeno pepper, sliced
- 4 Oz cream cheese
- Pepper
- Salt

Procedure:

1. Firstly, dd chicken, stock, jalapenos, and cream cheese into the instant pot.
2. Then, seal the pot with a lid and cook on high for 12 minutes.

3. Once done, release pressure using quick release. Remove lid.

4. Shred chicken using a fork.

5. Finally, set pot on sauté mode. Add remaining ingredients and stir well and cook until cheese is melted.

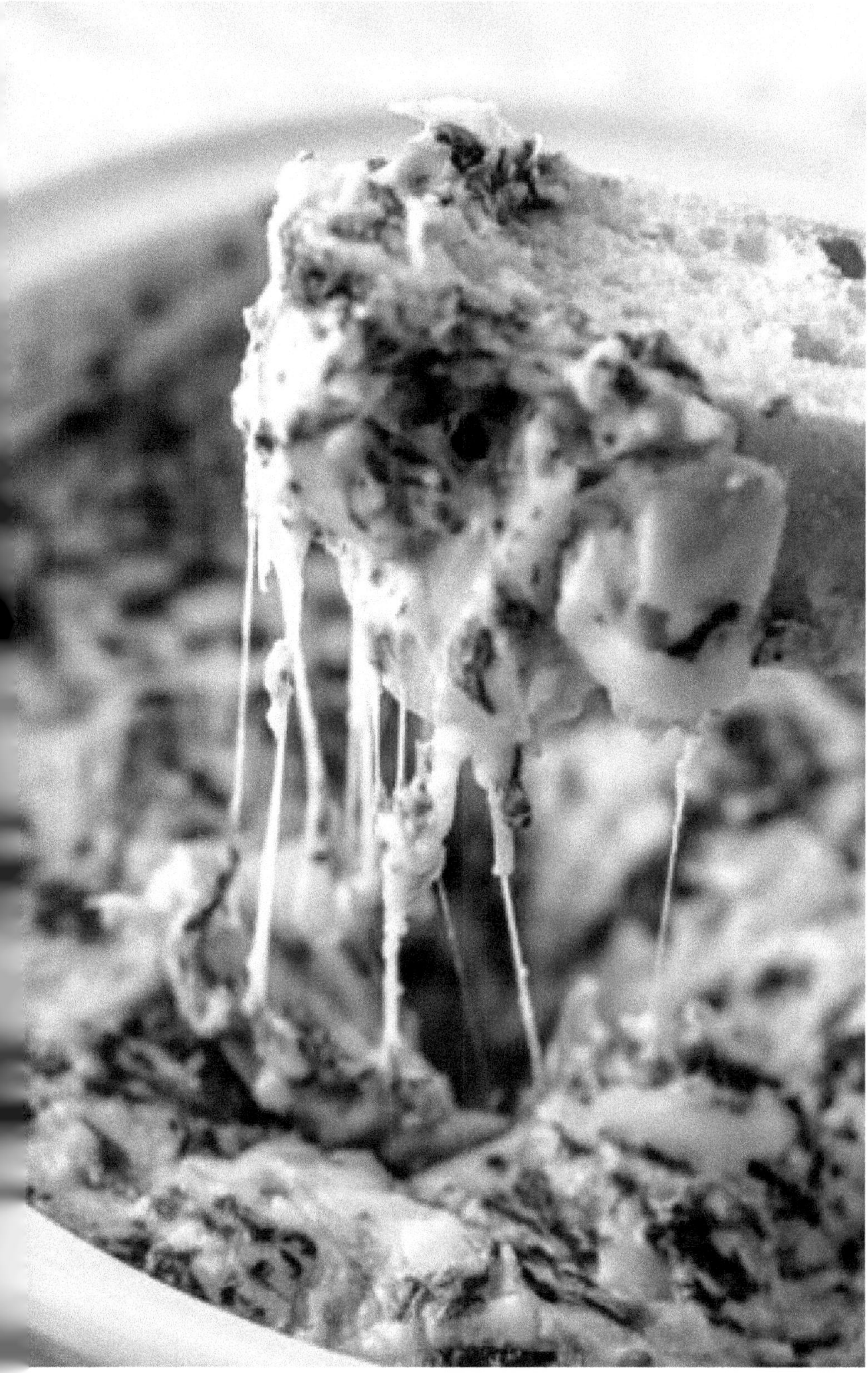

Slow Cooked Cheesy Artichoke Dip

Servings: 12

Preparation Time: 1 hour

Per Serving: Calories 226 Fat 19.3 g Carbohydrates 7.5 g Sugar 1.2 g Protein 6.8 g Cholesterol 51 mg

Ingredients:

- 20 Oz can artichoke hearts, drained and chopped
- 8 Cups spinach, chopped
- 16 Oz cream cheese
- 6 Tbsps sour cream
- 1/8 Cup mayonnaise
- 3/4 Cup mozzarella cheese, shredded
- 1/2 Cup parmesan cheese, grated
- 6 Garlic cloves, minced
- 1 Tsp dried parsley
- Pepper
- Salt

Procedure:

1. Firstly, add all ingredients into the inner pot of instant pot and stir well.
2. Then, seal the pot with the lid and select slow cook mode and set the timer for 60 minutes. Stir once while cooking.
3. Now, serve and enjoy.

Tasty Olive Eggplant Spread

Servings: 6

Preparation Time: 20 minutes

Per Serving: Calories 65 Fat 5.3 g Carbohydrates 4.7 g Sugar 2 g Protein 0.9 g Cholesterol 0 mg

Ingredients:

- 1 lb eggplant, chopped
- 1/4 Tbsp dried oregano
- 1/2 Cup olives, pitted and chopped
- 1/2 tbsp tahini
- 1/8 Cup fresh lime juice
- 1/4 Cup water
- 1 Garlic cloves
- 1/8 Cup olive oil
- Salt

Procedure:

1. Firstly, add oil into the inner pot of instant pot and set the pot on sauté mode.
2. Then, add eggplant and cook for 3-5 minutes.

3. Turn off sauté mode.

4. Add water and salt and stir well.

5. Finally, seal the pot with a lid and cook on high for 3 minutes.

6. Once done, release pressure using quick release. Remove lid.

7. Drain eggplant well and transfer into the food processor.

8. Add remaining ingredients into the food processor and process until smooth.

9. Now, serve and enjoy.

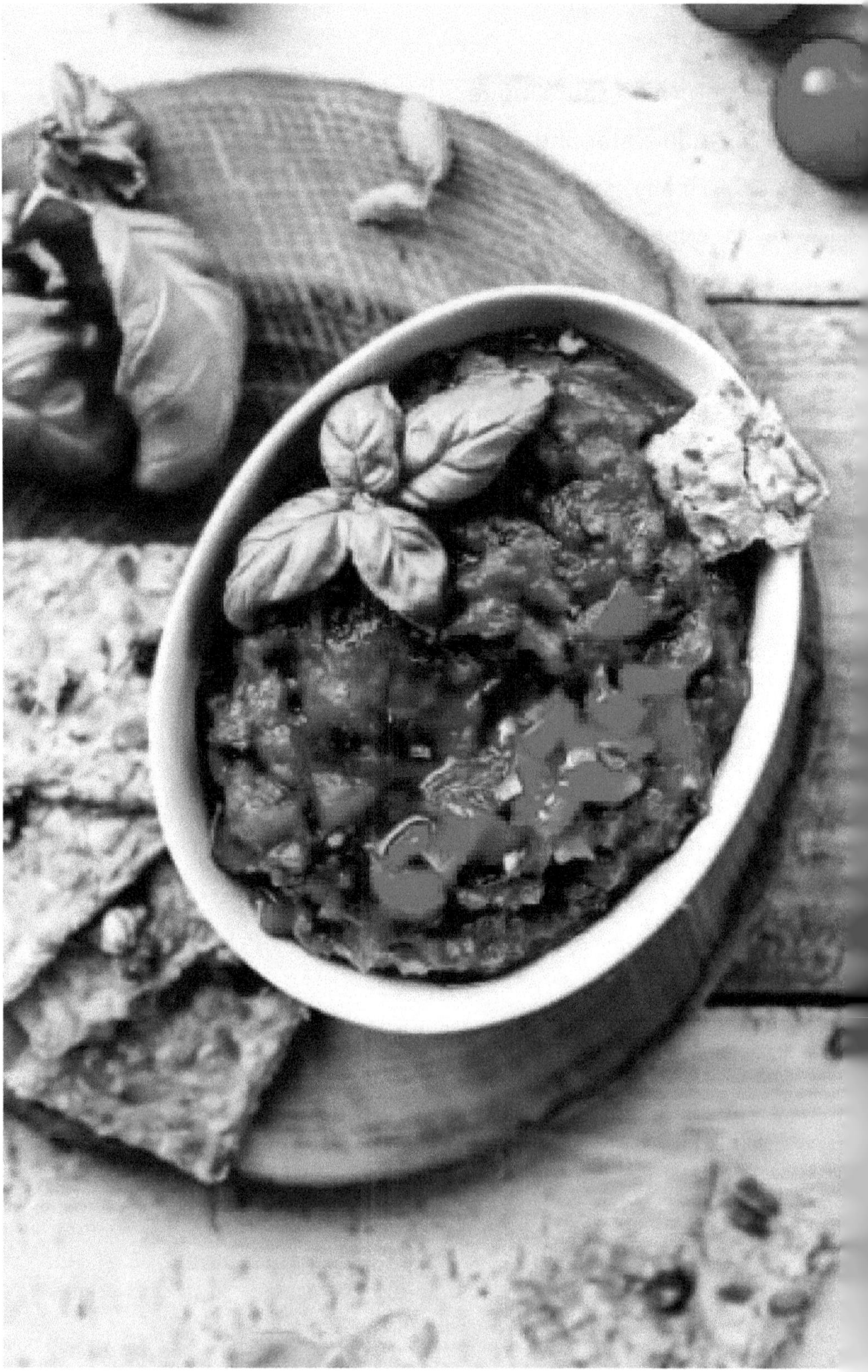

Enticing Pepper Tomato Eggplant Spread

Servings: 6

Preparation Time: 20 minutes

Per Serving: Calories 178 Fat 14.4 g Carbohydrates 12.8 g Sugar 7 g Protein 2.4 g Cholesterol 0 mg

Ingredients:

- 4 Cups eggplant, chopped
- 1/8 Cup vegetable broth
- 4 Tbsps tomato paste
- 1/2 Cup sun-dried tomatoes, minced
- 2 Cups bell pepper, chopped
- 2 Tsps garlic, minced
- 2 Cups onion, chopped
- 6 Tbsps olive oil
- Salt

Procedure:

1. Firstly, add oil into the inner pot of instant pot and set the pot on sauté mode.
2. Then, add onion and sauté for 3 minutes.

3. Add eggplant, bell pepper, and garlic and sauté for 2 minutes.
4. Finally, add the remaining ingredients and stir well.
5. Seal pot with lid and cook on high for 5 minutes.
6. Once done, release pressure using quick release. Remove lid.
7. Lightly mash the eggplant mixture using a potato masher.
8. Now, stir well and serve.

Delicious Healthy Spinach Dip

Servings: 8

Preparation Time: 10 minutes

Per Serving: Calories 109 Fat 9.2 g Carbohydrates 6.6 g Sugar 1.1 g Protein 3.2 g Cholesterol 0 mg

Ingredients:

- 28 Oz spinach
- 4 Tbsps fresh lime juice
- 2 Tbsps garlic, minced
- 4 Tbsps olive oil
- 4 Tbsps coconut cream
- Pepper
- Salt

Procedure:

1. First, add all ingredients except coconut cream into the instant pot and stir well.
2. Then, seal the pot with a lid and cook on low pressure for 8 minutes.

3. Once done, allow to release pressure naturally for 5 minutes, then release remaining using quick release. Remove lid.
4. Finally, add coconut cream and stir well and blend spinach mixture using a blender until smooth.
5. Now, serve and enjoy.

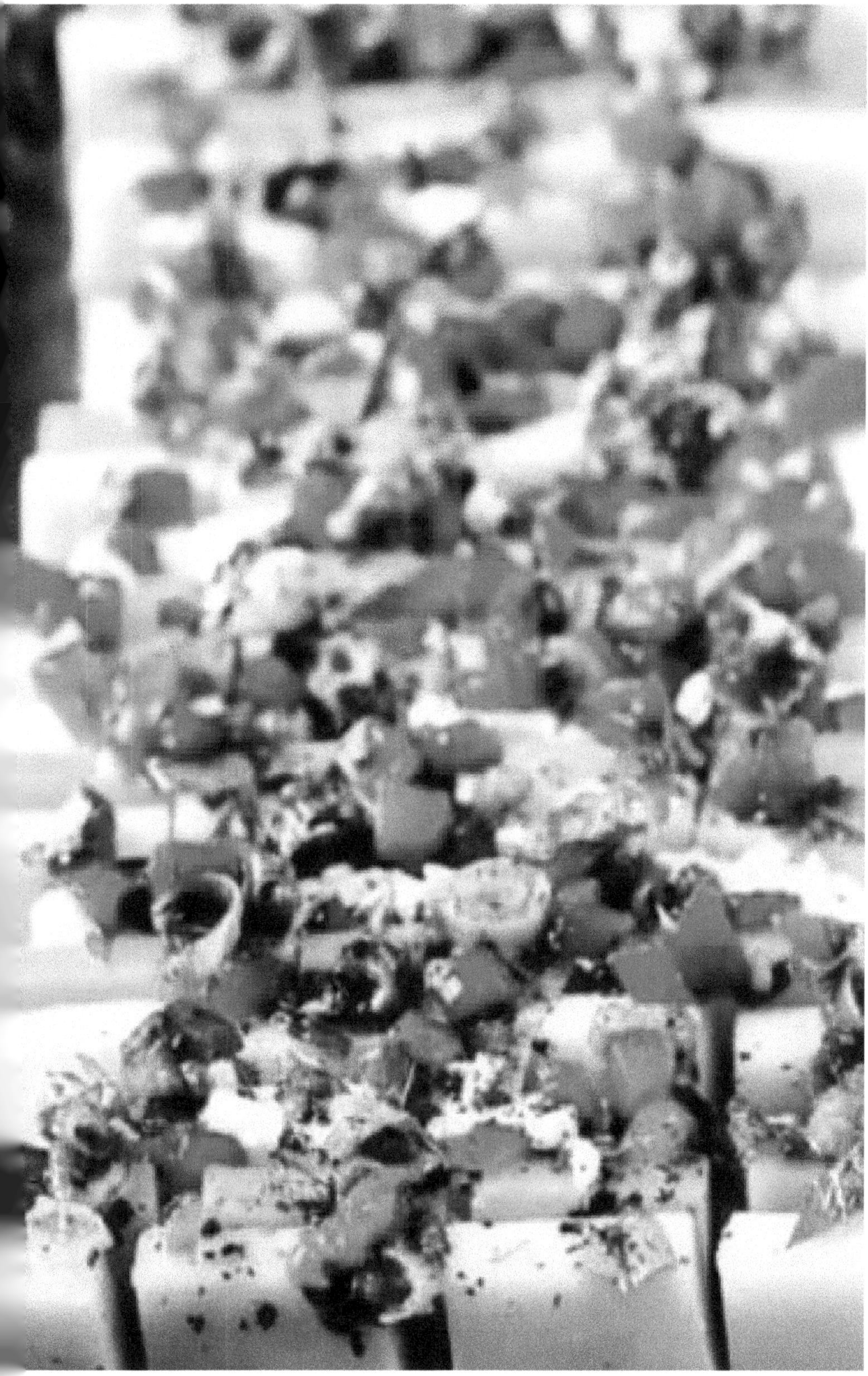

Tasty Marinated Cheese

Servings: 9

Preparation Time: 10 minutes

Per Serving: 44 cal., 4.3 g total fat (2.4 sat. fat), 13.9 mg chol., 40.6 mg sodium, 0.7 g total carbs., 0 g fiber, 0.4 g sugar, and 0.8 g protein

Ingredients:

- 4 Ounces cream cheese
- 3 Sprigs fresh thyme
- 1.1/2 Sprigs fresh rosemary
- 1 Garlic cloves, sliced
- 1/4 Cup sun-dried tomato vinaigrette dressing
- 1/2 Teaspoon black pepper
- 1/2 Lemon peel, cut into thin strips

Procedure:

1. First, cut the cream cheese into 36 cubes. Place on a serving tray.
2. Then, combine the remaining ingredients together.
3. Pour the dressing over the cheese; toss lightly.
4. Now, refrigerate for at least 1 hour to marinate.

Delectable Za'atar Fries

Servings: 10

Preparation Time: 35 minutes

Per Serving: calories 28, fat 2.9, fiber 0.2, carbs 0.6, protein 0.2

Ingredients:

- 2 Teaspoons Za'atar spices
- 6 Sweet potatoes
- 2 Tablespoons dried dill
- 2 Teaspoons salt
- 6 Teaspoons sunflower oil
- 1 Teaspoon paprika

Procedure:

1. Firstly, pour water in the crockpot. Peel the sweet potatoes and cut them into the fries.
2. Line the baking tray with parchment.
3. Then, place the layer of the sweet potato in the tray.
4. Sprinkle the vegetables with dried dill, salt, and paprika.

5. Finally, sprinkle sweet potatoes with Za'atar and mix up well with the help of the fingertips.
6. Sprinkle the sweet potato fries with sunflower oil.
7. Preheat the oven to 375F.
8. Now, bake the sweet potato fries for 35 minutes. Stir the fries every 10 minutes.

Tasty Tuna Salad

Servings: 8

Preparation Time: 10 minutes

Per Serving: 130 cal., 5 g total fat (0.5 g sat. fat), 25 mg chol., 240 mg sodium, 240 mg pot., 8 g total carbs., 1 g fiber, <1 g sugar, 12 g protein, 2% vitamin A, 2% vitamin C, 4% calcium, and 6% iron.

Ingredients:

- 2 Can (5 ounce) albacore tuna, solid white
- 1 to 4 Tablespoons mayo or Greek yogurt
- 2 Whole-wheat crackers (I used sleeve Ritz®)
- 1/8 Cup chickpeas, rinsed, drained (or preferred white beans)
- 1/2 Cup kalamata olives, quartered
- 1/2 Cup roughly chopped marinated artichoke hearts

Procedure:

1. Firstly, flake the tuna out of the can into a medium-sized bowl.

2. Then, add the chickpeas, olives, and artichoke hearts; toss to combine.
3. Add mayo or Greek yogurt according to your taste; stir until well combined.
4. Now, spoon the salad mixture onto crackers; serve.

Yummy Cucumber Gazpacho

Servings: 8

Preparation Time: 10 minutes

Per Serving: calories: 133 | fat: 1.5g | protein: 14.2g | carbs: 16.5g | fiber: 2.9g | sodium: 331mg

Ingredients:

- 4 Cucumbers, peeled, deseeded, and cut into chunks
- 1 Cup mint, finely chopped
- 4 Cups plain Greek yogurt
- 4 Garlic cloves, minced
- 4 Cups low-sodium vegetable soup
- 2 Tablespoon no-salt-added tomato paste
- 6 Teaspoons fresh dill
- Sea salt and freshly ground pepper, to taste

Procedure:

1. Firstly, put the cucumber, mint, yogurt, and garlic in a food processor, then pulse until creamy and smooth.

2. Transfer the puréed mixture in a large serving bowl, then add the vegetable soup, tomato paste, dill, salt, and ground black pepper. Stir to mix well.

3. Now, keep the soup in the refrigerator for at least 2 hours, then serve chilled.

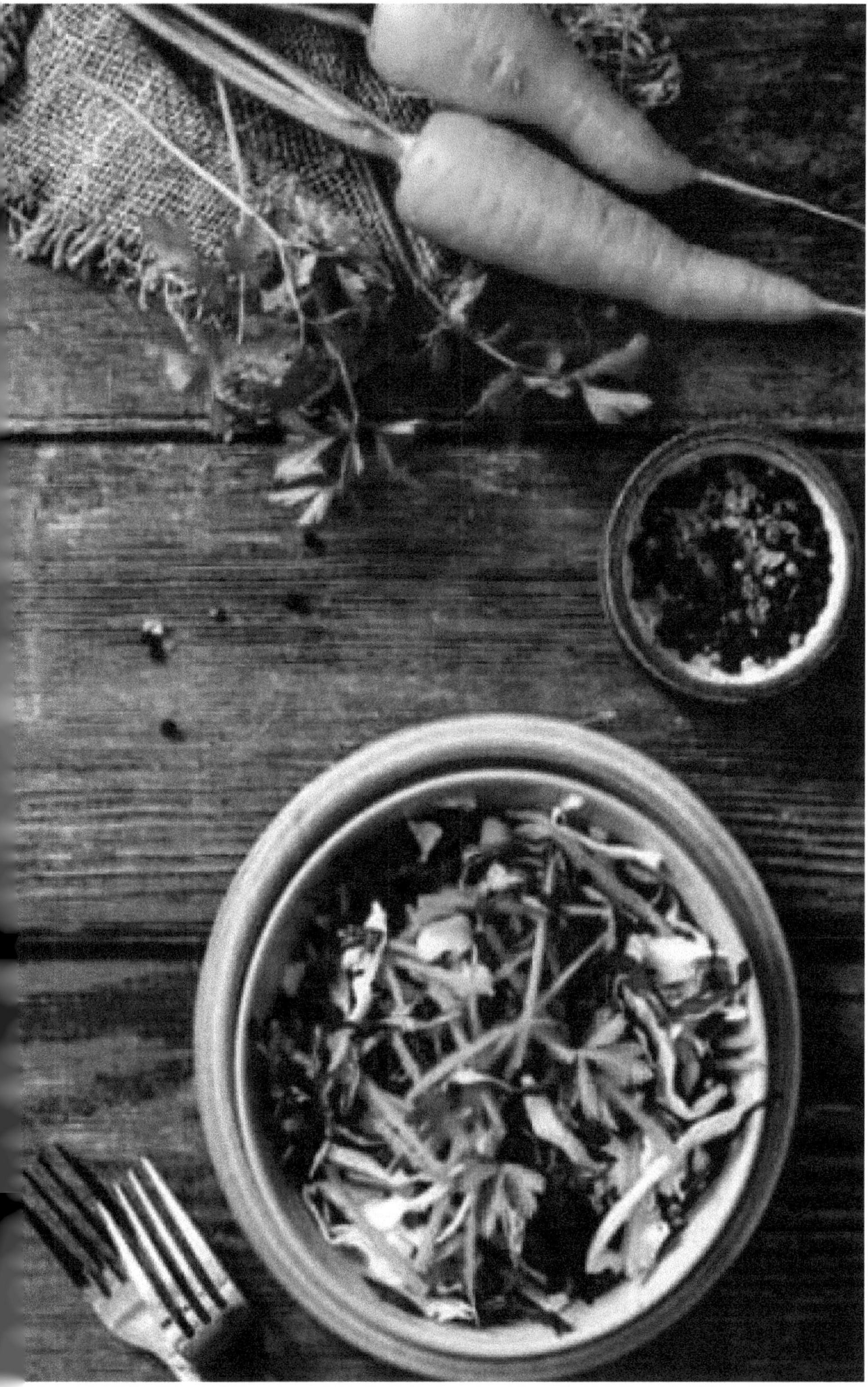

Easy Veggie Slaw

Servings: 12

Preparation Time: 20 minutes

Per Serving: calories: 387 | fat: 30.2g | protein: 8.1g | carbs: 25.9g | fiber: 6.0g | sodium: 980mg

Ingredients:

Salad:

- 4 Large broccoli stems, peeled and shredded
- 1 Celery root bulb, peeled and shredded
- 1/2 Cup chopped fresh Italian parsley
- 2 Large beets, peeled and shredded
- 4 Carrots, peeled and shredded
- 2 Small red onions, sliced thin
- 4 Zucchini, shredded

Dressing:

- 2 Teaspoons dijon mustard
- 1 Cup apple cider vinegar
- 2 Tablespoons raw honey
- 2 Teaspoons sea salt

- 1/2 Teaspoon freshly ground black pepper
- 4 Tablespoons extra-virgin olive oil

Topping:

- 1 Cup crumbled feta cheese

Procedure:

1. Firstly, combine the ingredients for the salad in a large salad bowl, then toss to combine well.
2. Then, combine the ingredients for the dressing in a small bowl, then stir to mix well.
3. Now, dress the salad, serve with feta cheese on top.

Yummy Grilled Bell Pepper and Anchovy Antipasto

Servings: 8

Preparation Time: 20 minutes

Per Serving: calories: 227 | fat: 14.9g | protein: 13.9g | carbs: 9.9g | fiber: 3.8g| sodium: 1913mg

Ingredients:

- 4 Tablespoons extra-virgin olive oil, divided
- 8 medium red bell peppers, quartered, stem and seeds removed
- 12 Ounces (170 g) anchovies in oil, chopped
- 4 Tablespoons capers, rinsed and drained
- 2 Cups Kalamata olives, pitted
- 2 Small shallots, chopped
- Sea salt and freshly ground pepper, to taste

Procedure:

1. Firstly, heat the grill to medium-high heat. Grease the grill grates with 1 tablespoon of olive oil.

2. Then, arrange the red bell peppers on the preheated grill grates, then grill for 8 minutes or until charred.
3. Finally, turn off the grill and allow the pepper to cool for 10 minutes.
4. Transfer the charred pepper in a colander. Rinse and peel the peppers under running cold water, then pat dry with paper towels.
5. Cut the peppers into chunks and combine them with the remaining ingredients in a large bowl. Toss to mix well.
6. Now, serve immediately.

Easy Root Vegetable Roast

Servings: 12

Preparation Time: 25 minutes

Per Serving: calories: 461 | fat: 18.1g | protein: 5.9g | carbs: 74.2g | fiber: 14.0g | sodium: 759mg

Ingredients:

- 2 Bunch beets, peeled and cut into 1-inch cubes
- 4 Small sweet potatoes, peeled and cut into 1-inch cubes
- 6 Parsnips, peeled and cut into 1-inch rounds
- 4 Carrots, peeled and cut into 1-inch rounds
- 2 Tablespoons raw honey
- 2 Teaspoons sea salt
- 1 Teaspoon freshly ground black pepper
- 2 Tablespoon extra-virgin olive oil
- 4 Tablespoons coconut oil, melted

Procedure:

1. Firstly, preheat the oven to 400ºF (205ºC). Line a baking sheet with parchment paper.

2. Then, combine all the ingredients in a large bowl. Toss to coat the vegetables well.
3. Pour the mixture in the baking sheet, then place the sheet in the preheated oven.
4. Roast for 25 minutes or until the vegetables are lightly browned and soft.
5. Finally, flip the vegetables halfway through the cooking time.
6. Now, remove the vegetables from the oven and allow to cool before serving.

SEAFOOD

Tasty Honey Balsamic Salmon

Servings: 4

Preparation Time: 10 minutes

Per Serving: Calories 303 Fat 11 g Carbohydrates 17.6 g Sugar 17.3 g Protein 34.6 g Cholesterol 78 mg

Ingredients:

- 4 Salmon fillets
- 1/2 Tsp red pepper flakes
- 4 Tbsps honey
- 4 Tbsps balsamic vinegar
- 2 Cups of water
- Pepper
- Salt

Procedure:

1. Firstly, pour water into the instant pot and place trivet in the pot.
2. Then, in a small bowl, mix together honey, red pepper flakes, and vinegar.

3. Brush fish fillets with honey mixture and place on top of the trivet.
4. Seal pot with lid and cook on high for 3 minutes.
5. Once done, release pressure using quick release. Remove lid.
6. Now, serve and enjoy.

Yummy Spicy Tomato Crab Mix

Servings: 8

Preparation Time: 20 minutes

Per Serving: Calories 142 Fat 5.7 g Carbohydrates 4.3 g Sugar 1.3 g Protein 14.7 g Cholesterol 61 mg

Ingredients:

- 2 lbs crab meat
- 2 Tsps paprika
- 1 Cup grape tomatoes, cut into half
- 4 Tbsps green onion, chopped
- 2 Tbsps olive oil
- Pepper
- Salt

Procedure:

1. Firstly, add oil into the inner pot of instant pot and set the pot on sauté mode.
2. Add paprika and onion and sauté for 2 minutes.
3. Then, add the rest of the ingredients and stir well.
4. Seal pot with lid and cook on high for 10 minutes.
5. Once done, release pressure using quick release. Remove lid.
6. Now, serve and enjoy.

Tempting Dill Halibut

Servings: 6

Preparation Time: 10 minutes

Per Serving: calories 170, fat 5.9, fiber 0.7, carbs 3.6, protein 25.1

Ingredients:

- 26 Oz halibut fillet
- 1/3 Cup cream
- 1/2 Cup dill, chopped
- 1 Teaspoon garlic powder
- 1/2 Teaspoon turmeric
- 1/2 teaspoon ground paprika
- 1/2 teaspoon salt
- 1/2 teaspoon olive oil

Procedure:

1. Firstly, chop the fish fillet on the big cubes and sprinkle them with garlic powder, turmeric, ground paprika, and salt.
2. Pour olive oil into the skillet and preheat it well.

3. Then, place fish in the hot oil and roast it for 2 minutes from each side over medium heat.
4. Add cream and stir gently with the help of the spatula.
5. Bring the mixture to boil and add dill.
6. Now, close the lid and cook fish on medium heat for 5 minutes.
7. Till the fish and creamy sauce are cooked.
8. Serve the halibut cubes with creamy sauce.

Tempting Salmon and Mango Mix

Servings: 4

Preparation Time: 25 minutes

Per Serving: calories 251, fat 15.9, fiber 5.9, carbs 26.4, protein 12.4

Ingredients:

- 4 Salmon fillets, skinless and boneless
- Salt and pepper to the taste
- 4 Tablespoons olive oil
- 2 Garlic cloves, minced
- 2 Mangos, peeled and cubed
- 2 Red chili, chopped
- 2 small piece gingers, grated
- Juice of 1 lime
- 1 tablespoon cilantro, chopped

Procedure:

1. Firstly, in a roasting pan, combine the salmon with the oil, garlic and the rest of the ingredients except the

cilantro, toss, introduce in the oven at 350 degrees F and bake for 25 minutes.

2. Then, divide everything between plates and serve with the cilantro sprinkled on top.

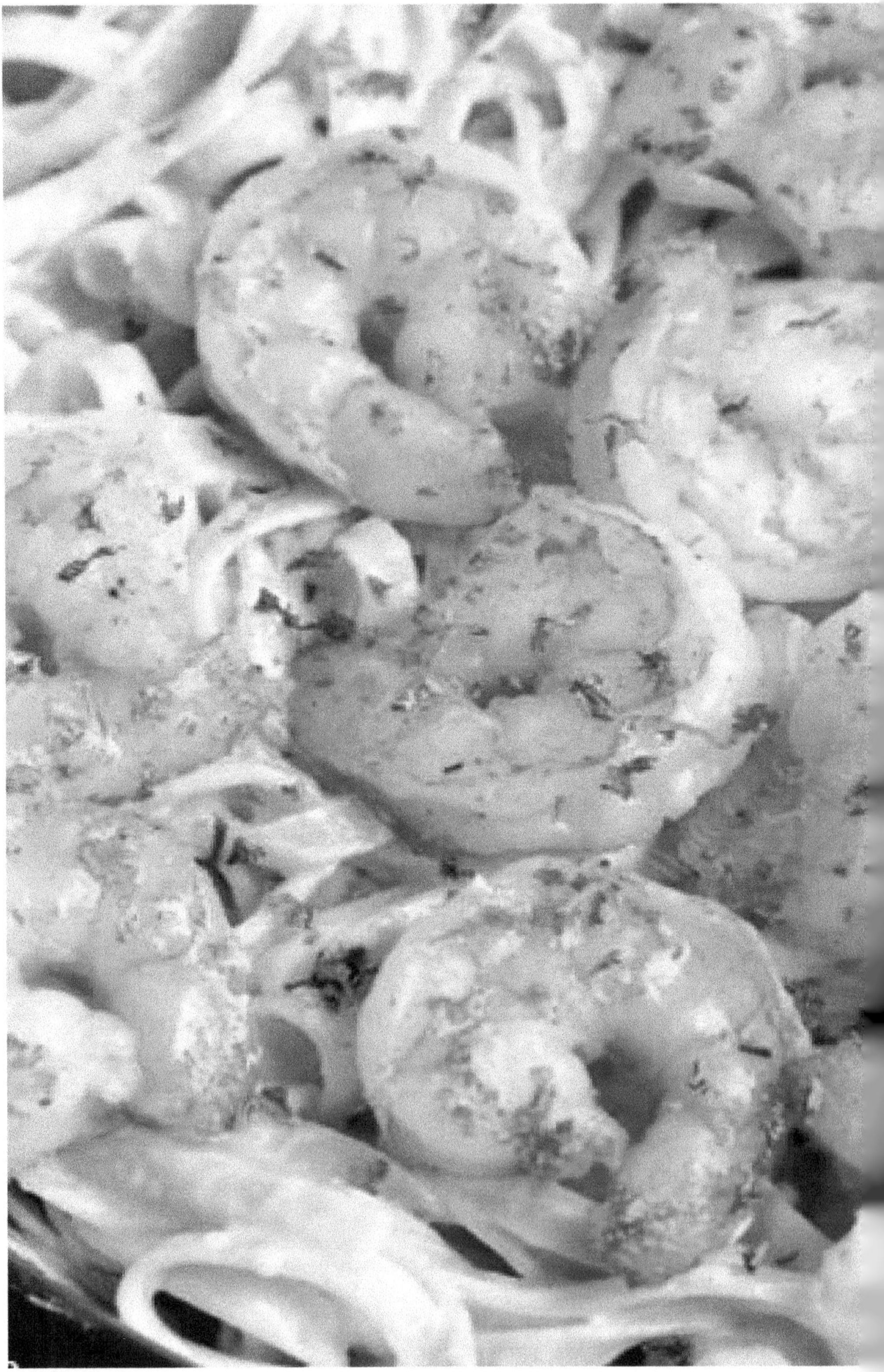

Delicious Shrimp Alfredo

Servings: 8

Preparation Time: 5 minutes

Per Serving: Calories 669 Fat 23.1 g Carbohydrates 76 g Sugar 2.4 g Protein 37.8 g Cholesterol 190 mg

Ingredients:

- 24 Shrimp, remove shells
- 1 tbsp garlic, minced
- 1/2 Cup parmesan cheese
- 4 Cups whole wheat rotini noodles
- 2 Cups fish broth
- 30 Oz alfredo sauce
- 1 Onion, chopped
- Salt

Procedure:

1. Firstly, add all ingredients except parmesan cheese into the instant pot and stir well.
2. Seal pot with lid and cook on high for 3 minutes.
3. Then, once done, release pressure using quick release. Remove lid.
4. Now, stir in cheese and serve.

Easy Cod and Mushrooms Mix

Servings: 8

Preparation Time: 50 minutes

Per Serving: calories 257, fat 10, fiber 3.1, carbs 24.3, protein 19.4

Ingredients:

- 4 Cod fillets, boneless
- 8 Tablespoons olive oil
- 8 Ounces mushrooms, sliced
- Sea salt and black pepper to the taste
- 24 cherry tomatoes, halved
- 16 Ounces lettuce leaves, torn
- 1 Avocado, pitted, peeled and cubed
- 1 Red chili pepper, chopped
- 1 Tablespoons cilantro, chopped
- 4 Tablespoons balsamic vinegar
- 2 Ounce feta cheese, crumbled

Procedure:

1. Firstly, put the fish in a roasting pan, brush it with 2 tablespoons oil, sprinkle salt and pepper all over and broil under medium-high heat for 15 minutes.
2. Meanwhile, heat up a pan with the rest of the oil over medium heat, add the mushrooms, stir and sauté for 5 minutes.
3. Then, add the rest of the ingredients, toss, cook for 5 minutes more and divide between plates.
4. Now, top with the fish and serve right away.

Tempting Baked Shrimp Mix

Servings: 8

Preparation Time: 30 minutes

Per Serving: calories 341, fat 19, fiber 9, carbs 34, protein 10

Ingredients:

- 8 Gold potatoes, peeled and sliced
- 2 Fennel bulbs, trimmed and cut into wedges
- 4 Shallots, chopped
- 4 Garlic cloves, minced
- 6 Tablespoons olive oil
- 1 Cup kalamata olives, pitted and halved
- 4 Pounds shrimp, peeled and deveined
- 2 Teaspoons lemon zest, grated
- 4 Teaspoons oregano, dried
- 8 Ounces feta cheese, crumbled
- 4 Tablespoons parsley, chopped

Procedure:

1. First, in a roasting pan, combine the potatoes with 2 tablespoons oil, garlic and the rest of the ingredients

except the shrimp, toss, introduce in the oven and bake at 450 degrees F for 25 minutes.

2. Then, add the shrimp, toss, bake for 7 minutes more, divide between plates and serve.

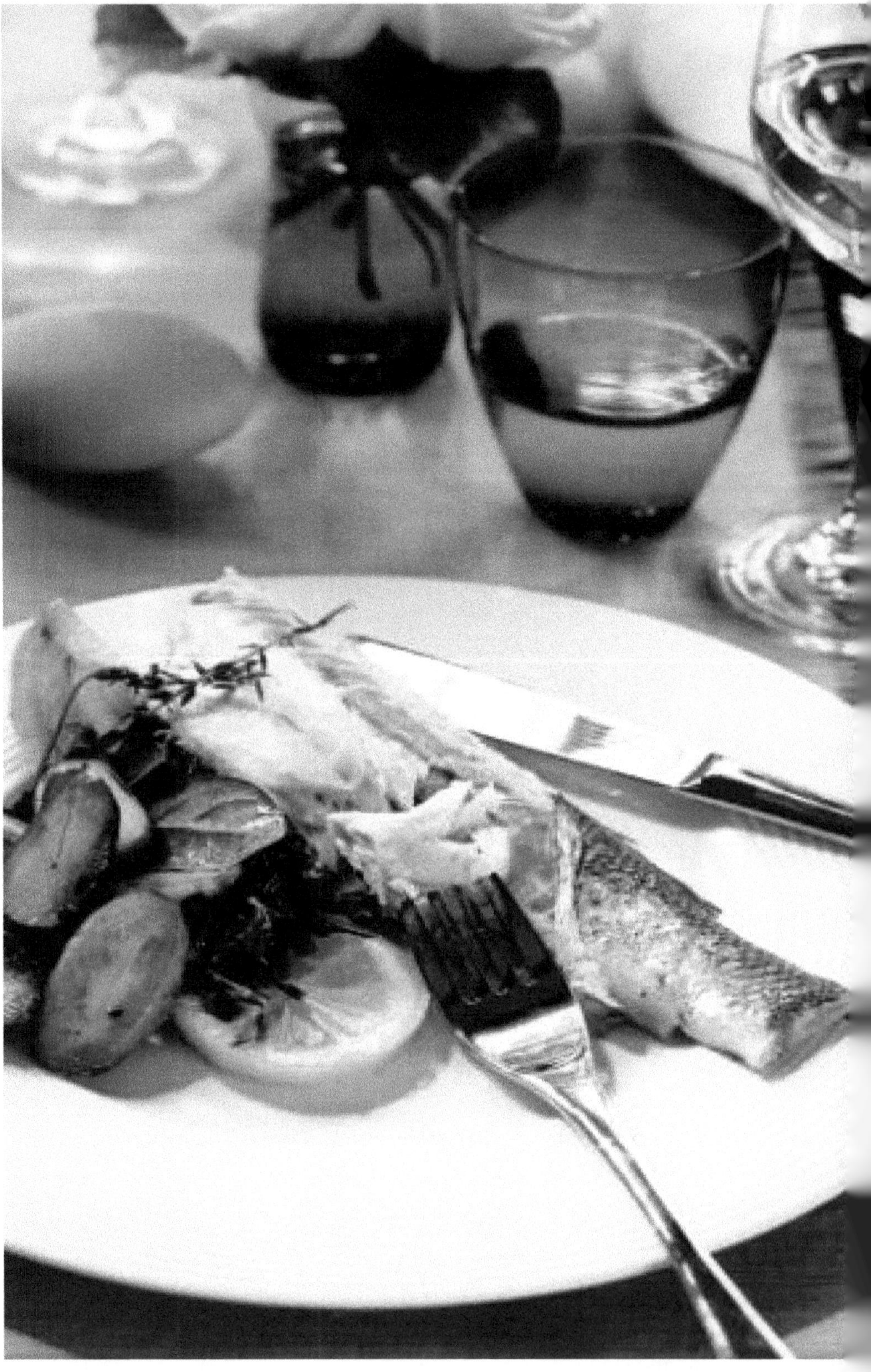

Pleasant Dill Baked Sea Bass

Servings: 12

Preparation Time: 25 minutes

Per Serving: calories: 224 | fat: 12.1g | protein: 28.1g | carbs: 0.9g | fiber: 0.3g | sodium: 104mg

Ingredients:

- 1 Cup olive oil
- 4 Pounds (907 g) sea bass
- Sea salt and freshly ground pepper, to taste
- 2 Garlic cloves, minced
- 1/2 Cup dry white wine
- 6 Teaspoons fresh dill
- 4 Teaspoons fresh thyme

Procedure:

1. Firstly, preheat the oven to 425ºF (220ºC).
2. Brush the bottom of a roasting pan with the olive oil. Place the fish in the pan and brush the fish with oil.

3. Then, season the fish with sea salt and freshly ground pepper. Combine the remaining ingredients and pour over the fish.
4. Bake in the preheated oven for 10 to 15 minutes, depending on the size of the fish.
5. Now, serve hot.

Delightful Sole Piccata with Cappe

Servings: 8

Preparation Time: 15 minutes

Per Serving: calories: 271 | fat:13.0g | protein: 30.0g | carbs: 7.0g | fiber: 0g | sodium: 413mg

Ingredients:

- 2 Teaspoons extra-virgin olive oil
- 8 (5-ounce / 142-g) sole fillets, patted dry
- 6 Tablespoons almond butter
- 4 Teaspoons minced garlic
- 4 Tablespoons all-purpose flour
- 4 Cups low-sodium chicken broth
- Juice and zest of ½ lemon
- 4 Tablespoons capers

Procedure:

1. Firstly, place a large skillet over medium-high heat and add the olive oil.
2. Sear the sole fillets until the fish flakes easily when tested with a fork, about 4 minutes on each side.

115

3. Then, transfer the fish to a plate and set it aside.

4. Return the skillet to the stove and add the butter.

5. Sauté the garlic until translucent, about 3 minutes.

6. Finally, whisk in the flour to make a thick paste and cook, stirring constantly, until the mixture is golden brown, about 2 minutes.

7. Whisk in the chicken broth, lemon juice and zest.

8. Cook for about 4 minutes until the sauce is thickened.

9. Now, stir in the capers and serve the sauce over the fish.

Tempting Haddock with Cucumber Sauce

Servings: 8

Preparation Time: 20 minutes

Per Serving: calories: 164 | fat: 2.0g | protein: 27.0g | carbs: 4.0g | fiber: 0g | sodium: 104mg

Ingredients:

- 1 Cup plain Greek yogurt
- 1 Scallion, white and green parts, finely chopped
- 1 English cucumber, grated, liquid squeezed out
- 4 Teaspoons chopped fresh mint
- 2 Teaspoons honey
- Sea salt and freshly ground black pepper, to taste
- 8 (5-ounce / 142-g) haddock fillets, patted dry
- Non-stick cooking spray

Procedure

1. Firstly, in a small bowl, stir together the yogurt, cucumber, scallion, mint, honey, and a pinch of salt. Set aside.
2. Then, season the fillets lightly with salt and pepper.

3. Place a large skillet over medium-high heat and spray lightly with cooking spray.
4. Cook the haddock, turning once until it is just cooked through, about 5 minutes per side.
5. Finally, remove the fish from the heat and transfer it to plates. Serve topped with the cucumber sauce.

Pleasant Crispy Herb Crusted Halibut

Servings: 8

Preparation Time: 30 minutes

Per Serving: calories: 262 | fat: 11.0g | protein: 32.0g | carbs: 4.0g | fiber: 2.0g | sodium: 77mg

Ingredients:

- 8 (5-ounce / 142-g) halibut fillets, patted dry
- Extra-virgin olive oil, for brushing
- 1 Cup coarsely ground unsalted pistachios
- 2 Tablespoons chopped fresh parsley
- 2 Teaspoons chopped fresh basil
- 2 Teaspoons chopped fresh thyme
- Pinch sea salt
- Pinch freshly ground black pepper

Procedure:

1. Firstly, preheat the oven to 350ºF (180ºC). Line a baking sheet with parchment paper.
2. Place the fillets on the baking sheet and brush them generously with olive oil.

3. Then, in a small bowl, stir together the pistachios, parsley, basil, thyme, salt, and pepper.
4. Spoon the nut mixture evenly on the fish, spreading it out so the tops of the fillets are covered.
5. Finally, bake in the preheated oven until it flakes when pressed with a fork, about 20 minutes.
6. Now, serve immediately.

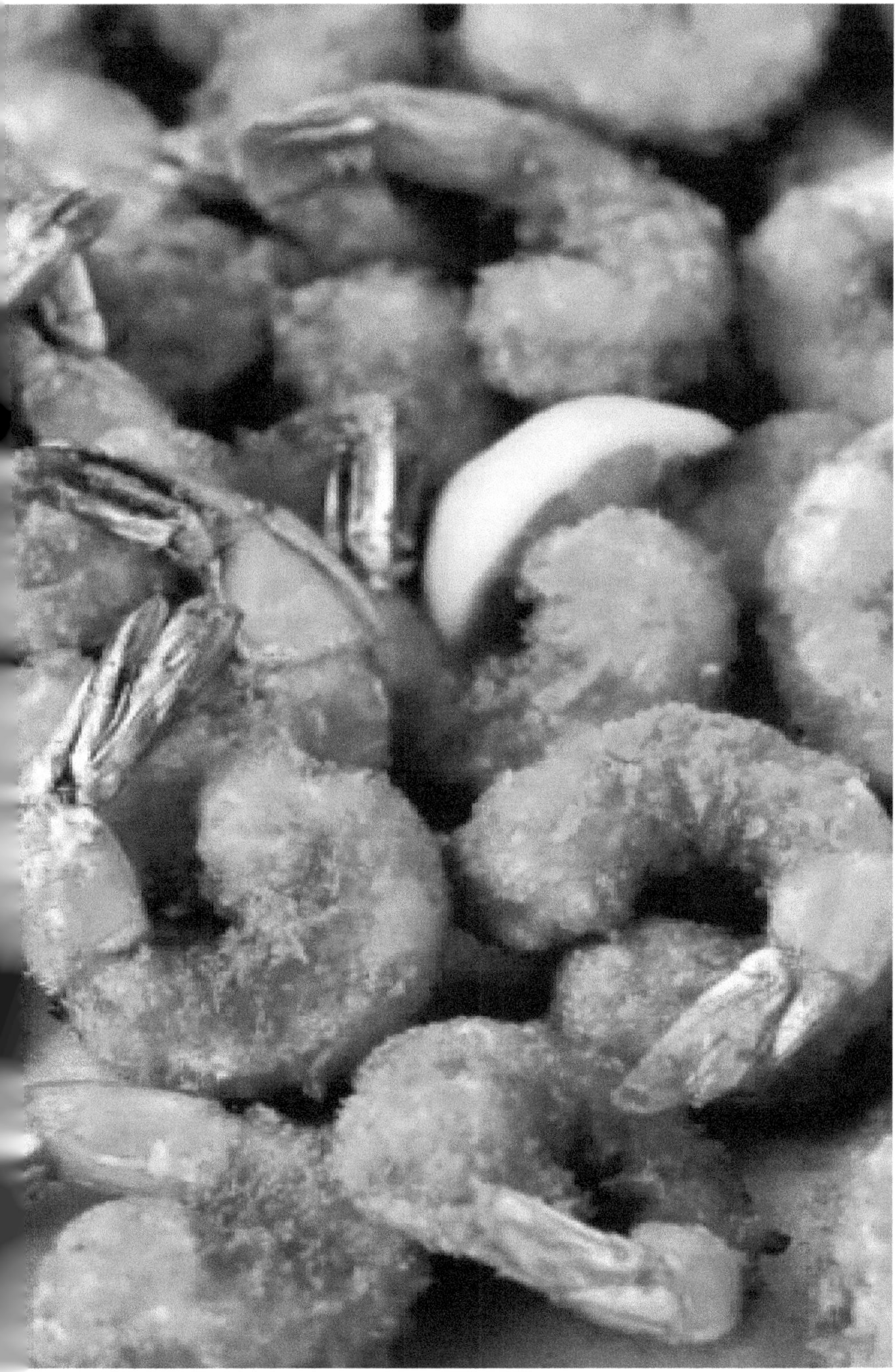

Flavorful Breaded Shrimp

Servings: 8

Preparation Time: 10 minutes

Per Serving: calories: 714 | fat: 34.0g | protein: 37.0g | carbs: 63.0g | fiber: 3.0g | sodium: 1727mg

Ingredients:

- 4 Large eggs
- 1 Tablespoon water
- 4 Cups seasoned Italian bread crumbs
- 2 Teaspoons salt
- 2 Cups flour
- 2 Pounds (454 g) large shrimp (21 to 25), peeled and deveined
- Extra-virgin olive oil, as needed

Procedure:

1. Firstly, in a small bowl, beat the eggs with the water, then transfer to a shallow dish.
2. Add the bread crumbs and salt to a separate shallow dish, then mix well.

3. Place the flour into a third shallow dish.

4. Coat the shrimp in the flour, then the beaten egg, and finally the bread crumbs. Place on a plate and repeat with all of the shrimp.

5. Then, heat a skillet over high heat.

6. Pour in enough olive oil to coat the bottom of the skillet.

7. Finally, cook the shrimp in the hot skillet for 2 to 3 minutes on each side. Remove and drain on a paper towel.

8. Now, serve warm.

Lightning Source UK Ltd.
Milton Keynes UK
UKHW020650210521
384114UK00001B/106